Concise Medicine: Clinical Pearls and Algorithms in Internal Medicine

Printed in the United States of America

Library of Congress Cataloging-in-Publication data available on request from the publisher.

ISBN: 978-0-578-56951-2

Cover Design by Oladimeji

For more information contact:

Nicholas Hatcher

http://www.Nurse-Doctor.com

Table of Contents

Preface

As a student navigating my way through volumes of content to eventually become a healthcare provider, I recognized the importance of having easily accessible, organized, and concise reference content to provide high-quality, evidence-based, and cost-effective care. Many pocket references provide lists and paragraphs with little visual content to aid the reader in the construction of a differential diagnosis and treatment plan. Other books aiding in this endeavor are beautifully written but are too large and cumbersome to carry to a practice site.

One of the most influential statements made by a mentor was to "keep a practice notebook". This practice notebook grew from a small hand-written book with some scattered images and tables to the book you hold now. During the early process of developing my practice notebook I was able to identify a cognitive process integral to the clinician's ability to diagnose, pattern recognition. Through independent study, I explored methods of operationalizing this cognitive process. After personal experimentation in the practice setting, I ultimately determined that the most effective method of mobilizing pattern recognition is through algorithms. I then worked to convert all of my notes from books, journals, lectures, and conferences into algorithmic form in an effort to show the movement through key steps in working through differential diagnoses. During this process, my work was recognized by a handful of colleagues, who recommended dissemination of my work.

Now, after four years of adding, refining, and editing while personally implementing the content of my book in my primary role as a hospitalist, I have completed the first edition of Concise Medicine. Concise medicine features over 150 algorithms and over 50 images with scattered clinical pearls designed for the student and practicing clinician. Concise Medicine emphasizes essential steps needed to arrive at a diagnosis and treatment plan. Unlike many existing references, Concise Medicine remains as the book title suggests and remains visually oriented and to-the-point.

About the Author

Dr. Nicholas Hatcher is a Doctor of Nursing Practice and board-certified adult-gerontology acute care nurse practitioner. He achieved his Master of Science in Nursing degree in 2016 and became a Doctor of Nursing Practice in 2018. He started his educational career at Cleveland State Community College School of Nursing in Cleveland, Tennessee, where he achieved his Associate Degree in Nursing. He then went to Vanderbilt University School of Nursing in Nashville, Tennessee, where he achieved his Bachelor of Science in Nursing, Master of Science in Nursing, and Doctor of Nursing Practice Degrees. Dr. Hatcher enjoys approaching patients using a biopsychosocial model, which was his original inspiration for the nursing profession. To further develop this approach, Dr. Hatcher is currently attending a post-degree Psychiatric Mental Health Nurse Practitioner program at John's Hopkins University School of Nursing. Dr. Hatcher's primary practice role is as an internal medicine hospitalist with secondary roles in inpatient and outpatient psychiatry as well as education. Dr. Hatcher enjoys spending time with his wife, Sarah Hatcher, and son, Damian Hatcher, who are both a great source of inspiration for his work. In his leisure, Dr. Hatcher enjoys reading medical literature, creating medical art, and designing educational material.

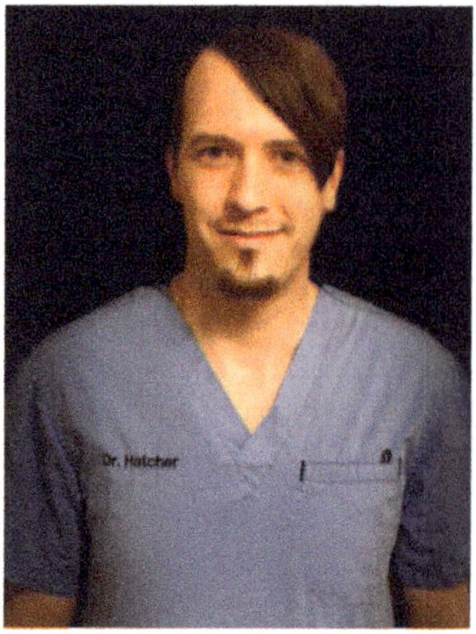

Constitutional Manifestations

Night Sweats

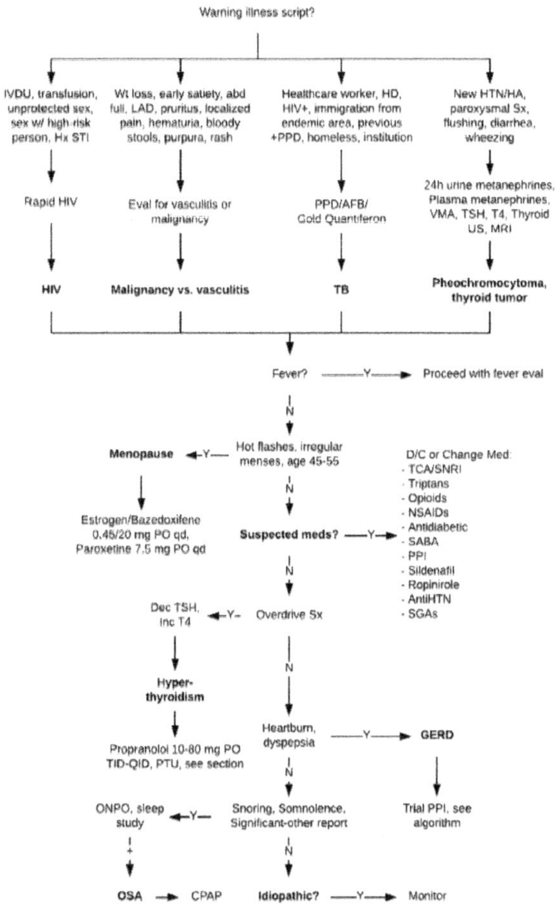

Fever

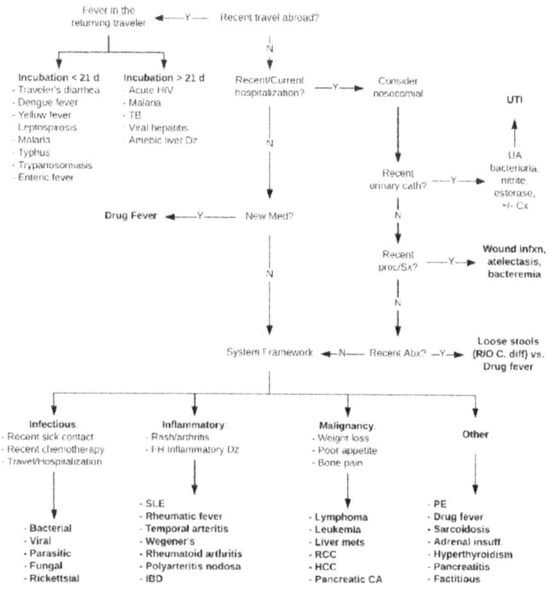
Fever in the returning traveler
Y
Recent travel abroad?
N
Incubation < 21 d
- Traveler's diarrhea
- Dengue fever
- Yellow fever
- Leptospirosis
- Malaria
- Typhus
- Trypanosomiasis
- Enteric fever
Incubation > 21 d
- Acute HIV
- Malaria
- TB
- Viral hepatitis
- Amebic liver Dz
Recent/Current hospitalization?
Y
Consider nosocomial
UTI
N
UA bacteriuria, nitrite, esterase, +/- Cx
Recent urinary cath?
Y
N
Drug Fever
Y
New Med?
N
Recent proc/Sx?
Y
Wound infxn, atelectasis, bacteremia
N
System Framework
N
Recent Abx?
Y
Loose stools (R/O C. diff) vs. Drug fever
Infectious
- Recent sick contact
- Recent chemotherapy
- Travel/Hospitalization
Inflammatory
- Rash/arthritis
- FH Inflammatory Dz
Malignancy
- Weight loss
- Poor appetite
- Bone pain
Other
- Bacterial
- Viral
- Parasitic
- Fungal
- Rickettsial
- SLE
- Rheumatic fever
- Temporal arteritis
- Wegener's
- Rheumatoid arthritis
- Polyarteritis nodosa
- IBD
- Lymphoma
- Leukemia
- Liver mets
- RCC
- HCC
- Pancreatic CA
- PE
- Drug fever
- Sarcoidosis
- Adrenal insuff.
- Hyperthyroidism
- Pancreatitis
- Factitious

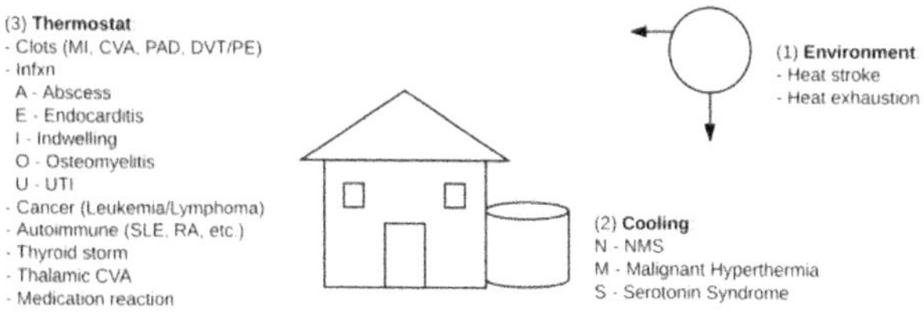
(3) Thermostat
- Clots (MI, CVA, PAD, DVT/PE)
- Infxn
A - Abscess
E - Endocarditis
I - Indwelling
O - Osteomyelitis
U - UTI
- Cancer (Leukemia/Lymphoma)
- Autoimmune (SLE, RA, etc.)
- Thyroid storm
- Thalamic CVA
- Medication reaction
(1) Environment
- Heat stroke
- Heat exhaustion
(2) Cooling
N - NMS
M - Malignant Hyperthermia
S - Serotonin Syndrome

Fatigue

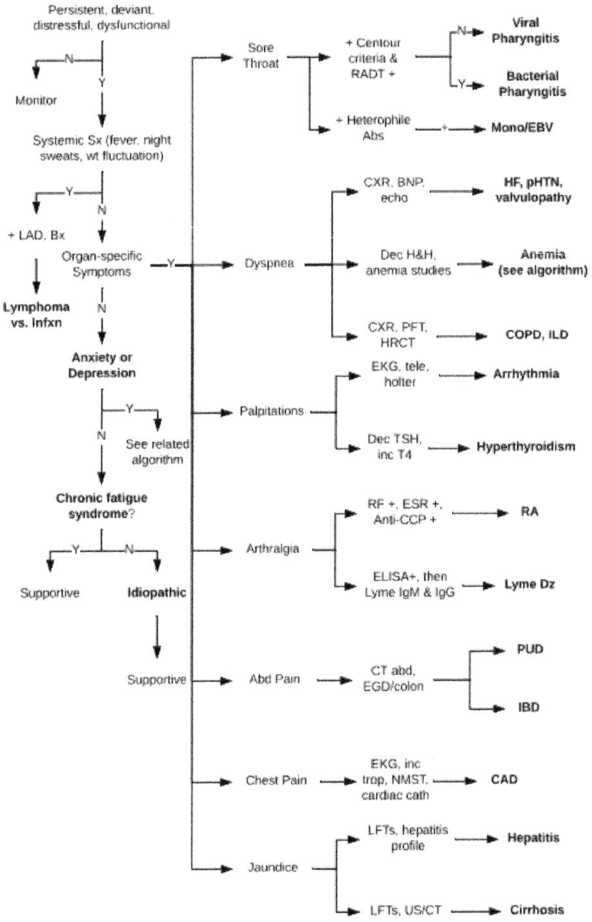
Persistent, deviant, distressful, dysfunctional
N
Y
Monitor
Systemic Sx (fever, night sweats, wt fluctuation)
Y
N
+ LAD, Bx
Lymphoma vs. Infxn
Organ-specific Symptoms
Y
N
Anxiety or Depression
Y
N
See related algorithm
Chronic fatigue syndrome?
Y
N
Supportive
Idiopathic
Supportive
Sore Throat
+ Centour criteria & RADT +
N
Viral Pharyngitis
Y
Bacterial Pharyngitis
+ Heterophile Abs
+
Mono/EBV
Dyspnea
CXR, BNP, echo
HF, pHTN, valvulopathy
Dec H&H, anemia studies
Anemia (see algorithm)
CXR, PFT, HRCT
COPD, ILD
Palpitations
EKG, tele, holter
Arrhythmia
Dec TSH, inc T4
Hyperthyroidism
Arthralgia
RF +, ESR +, Anti-CCP +
RA
ELISA+, then Lyme IgM & IgG
Lyme Dz
Abd Pain
CT abd, EGD/colon
PUD
IBD
Chest Pain
EKG, inc trop, NMST, cardiac cath
CAD
Jaundice
LFTs, hepatitis profile
Hepatitis
LFTs, US/CT
Cirrhosis

Weight Gain

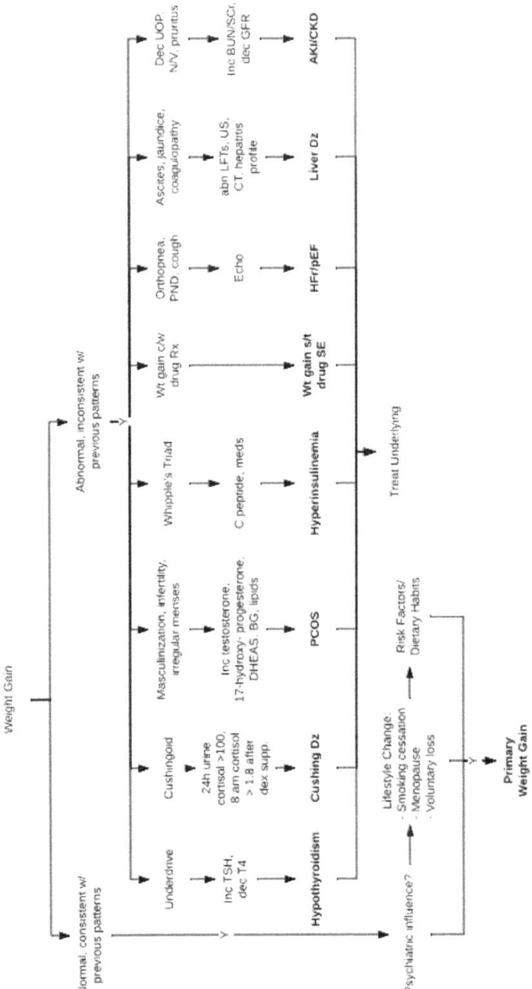

Weight Gain
Normal, consistent w/ previous patterns
Abnormal, inconsistent w/ previous patterns
Y
Underdrive
Inc TSH, dec T4
Hypothyroidism
Cushingoid
24h urine cortisol >100, 8 am cortisol > 1.8 after dex supp.
Cushing Dz
Masculinization, infertility, irregular menses
Inc testosterone, 17-hydroxy- progesterone, DHEAS, BG, lipids
PCOS
Whipple's Triad
C peptide, meds
Hyperinsulinemia
Wt gain c/w drug Rx
Wt gain s/t drug SE
Orthopnea, PND, cough
Echo
HFr/pEF
Ascites, jaundice, coagulopathy
abn LFTs, US, CT, hepatitis profile
Liver Dz
Dec UOP, N/V, pruritus
Inc BUN/SCr, dec GFR
AKI/CKD
Treat Underlying
Psychiatric influence?
Lifestyle Change:
· Smoking cessation
· Menopause
· Voluntary loss
Risk Factors/ Dietary Habits
Primary Weight Gain

Weight Loss

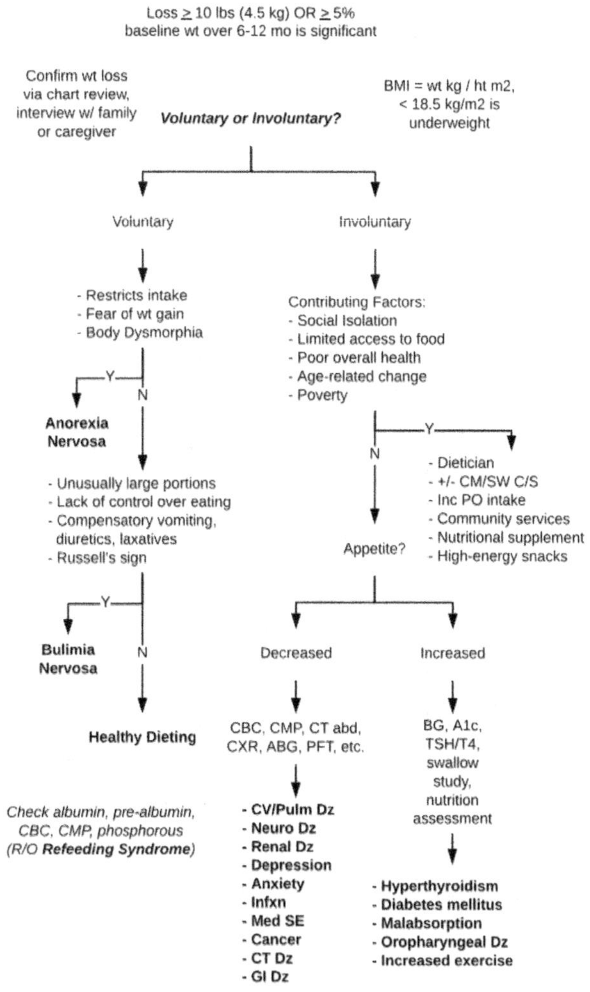
Loss ≥ 10 lbs (4.5 kg) OR ≥ 5% baseline wt over 6-12 mo is significant
Confirm wt loss via chart review, interview w/ family or caregiver
Voluntary or Involuntary?
BMI = wt kg / ht m2, < 18.5 kg/m2 is underweight
Voluntary
Involuntary
- Restricts intake
- Fear of wt gain
- Body Dysmorphia
Y
N
Anorexia Nervosa
- Unusually large portions
- Lack of control over eating
- Compensatory vomiting, diuretics, laxatives
- Russell's sign
Y
N
Bulimia Nervosa
Healthy Dieting
Check albumin, pre-albumin, CBC, CMP, phosphorous (R/O Refeeding Syndrome)
Contributing Factors:
- Social Isolation
- Limited access to food
- Poor overall health
- Age-related change
- Poverty
Y
N
- Dietician
- +/- CM/SW C/S
- Inc PO intake
- Community services
- Nutritional supplement
- High-energy snacks
Appetite?
Decreased
Increased
CBC, CMP, CT abd, CXR, ABG, PFT, etc.
- CV/Pulm Dz
- Neuro Dz
- Renal Dz
- Depression
- Anxiety
- Infxn
- Med SE
- Cancer
- CT Dz
- GI Dz
BG, A1c, TSH/T4, swallow study, nutrition assessment
- Hyperthyroidism
- Diabetes mellitus
- Malabsorption
- Oropharyngeal Dz
- Increased exercise

Insomnia

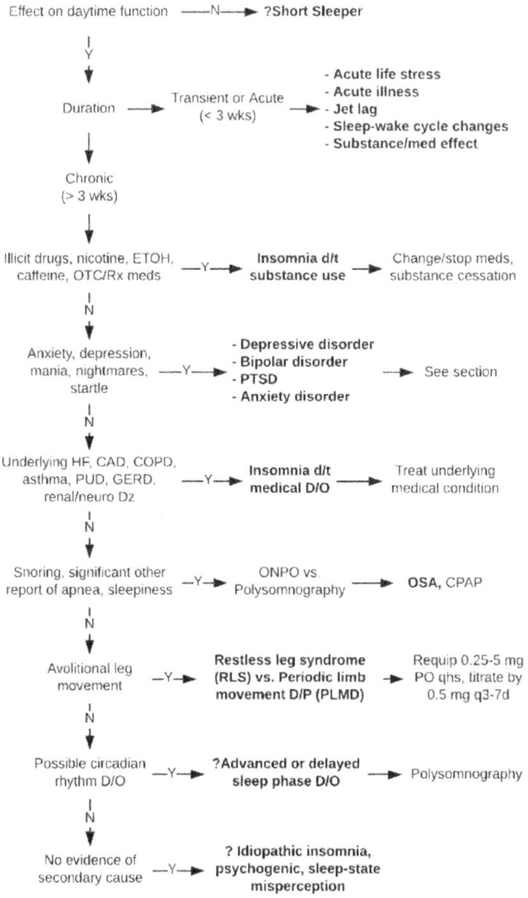
Effect on daytime function
N
?Short Sleeper
Y
Duration
Transient or Acute (< 3 wks)
- Acute life stress
- Acute illness
- Jet lag
- Sleep-wake cycle changes
- Substance/med effect
Chronic (> 3 wks)
Illicit drugs, nicotine, ETOH, caffeine, OTC/Rx meds
Y
Insomnia d/t substance use
Change/stop meds, substance cessation
N
Anxiety, depression, mania, nightmares, startle
Y
- Depressive disorder
- Bipolar disorder
- PTSD
- Anxiety disorder
See section
N
Underlying HF, CAD, COPD, asthma, PUD, GERD, renal/neuro Dz
Y
Insomnia d/t medical D/O
Treat underlying medical condition
N
Snoring, significant other report of apnea, sleepiness
Y
ONPO vs. Polysomnography
OSA, CPAP
N
Avolitional leg movement
Y
Restless leg syndrome (RLS) vs. Periodic limb movement D/P (PLMD)
Requip 0.25-5 mg PO qhs, titrate by 0.5 mg q3-7d
N
Possible circadian rhythm D/O
Y
?Advanced or delayed sleep phase D/O
Polysomnography
N
No evidence of secondary cause
Y
? Idiopathic insomnia, psychogenic, sleep-state misperception

Neurology

Altered Mental Status (AMS)

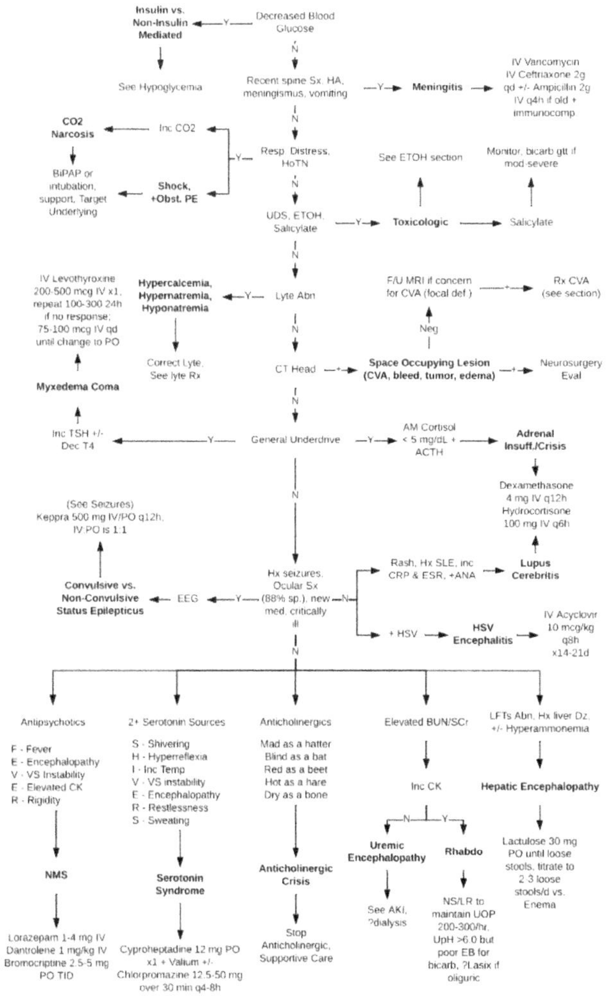

Syncope

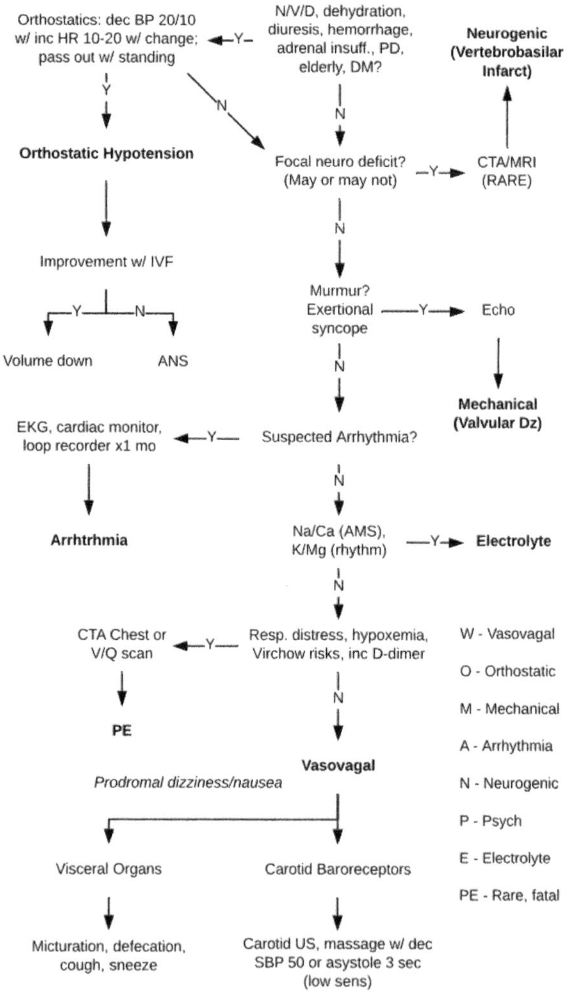

Orthostatics: dec BP 20/10 w/ inc HR 10-20 w/ change; pass out w/ standing
Y
N/V/D, dehydration, diuresis, hemorrhage, adrenal insuff., PD, elderly, DM?
Neurogenic (Vertebrobasilar Infarct)
Y
N
N
Orthostatic Hypotension
Focal neuro deficit? (May or may not)
Y
CTA/MRI (RARE)
N
Improvement w/ IVF
Y
N
Volume down
ANS
Murmur? Exertional syncope
Y
Echo
N
Mechanical (Valvular Dz)
EKG, cardiac monitor, loop recorder x1 mo
Y
Suspected Arrhythmia?
N
Arrhtrhmia
Na/Ca (AMS), K/Mg (rhythm)
Y
Electrolyte
N
CTA Chest or V/Q scan
Y
Resp. distress, hypoxemia, Virchow risks, inc D-dimer
N
PE
Vasovagal
Prodromal dizziness/nausea
Visceral Organs
Carotid Baroreceptors
Micturation, defecation, cough, sneeze
Carotid US, massage w/ dec SBP 50 or asystole 3 sec (low sens)
W - Vasovagal
O - Orthostatic
M - Mechanical
A - Arrhythmia
N - Neurogenic
P - Psych
E - Electrolyte
PE - Rare, fatal

Seizure

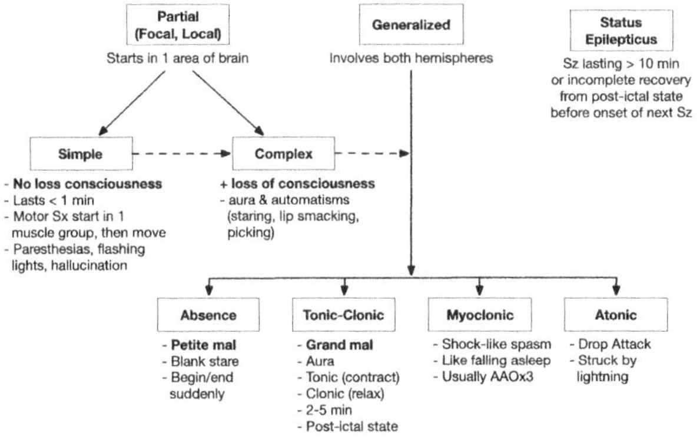

Etiology:

S – Substrates (sugar, O2)

I – Isoniazid OD

C – Cations (Na, Ca, Mg)

K – Kids (eclampsia)

D – Drugs (CRAP: Cocaine, Rum, Amphetamines, PCP)

R – Rum (Alcohol W/D – also BZD W/D)

I – Illness (chronic Sz D/O et al. chronic D/O)

F – Fever (esp. child; meningitis, encephalitis, abscess)

T – Trauma (CVD, EDH, SDH, IPH)

E – Extra toxicologic
- TAIL: Theophylline, ASA, Isoniazid, Lithium
- 3 Anti's: Antihistamine OD, Antidepressant OD, Anticonvulsants (too high Dilantin/Tegretol)

R – Rat poison (organophosphate poisoning)

Management (by minute):

0: Rapid ABC, VS, BG

1: Lorazepam 2 mg IV (avg. Sz)
Diazepam 5-10 mg IV (status)

2: SpO2 mon, EKG, IV x1, BMP, Ca, Mg, PO4-, LFTs, AED levels, ABG, UDS

5: Thiamine 100 mg IV then D50 push, lorazepam 0.1 mg/kg IV (<2 mg/min)

10: Choose one:
- Keppra 50 mg/kg IV
- PHT load 20 mg/kg, then 50 mg/min. Send PHT level 20 min after loading dose (18-30 mg/L).
- Depakote 30 mg/kg IV (VPA level 70-120 mg/mL)

30: Phenobarbital 75 mg/min (level 25-50 mg/L)

50: Intubate, continuous EEG
- Midazolam 0.2 mg/kg IV load, then 0.1-0.4 mg/kg/hr
- Propofol 1-2 mg/kg load, then 2-10 mg/kg/hr

60+: Check levels, adjust meds per EEG, taper off, CT head, f/u MRI/EEG

Vertigo

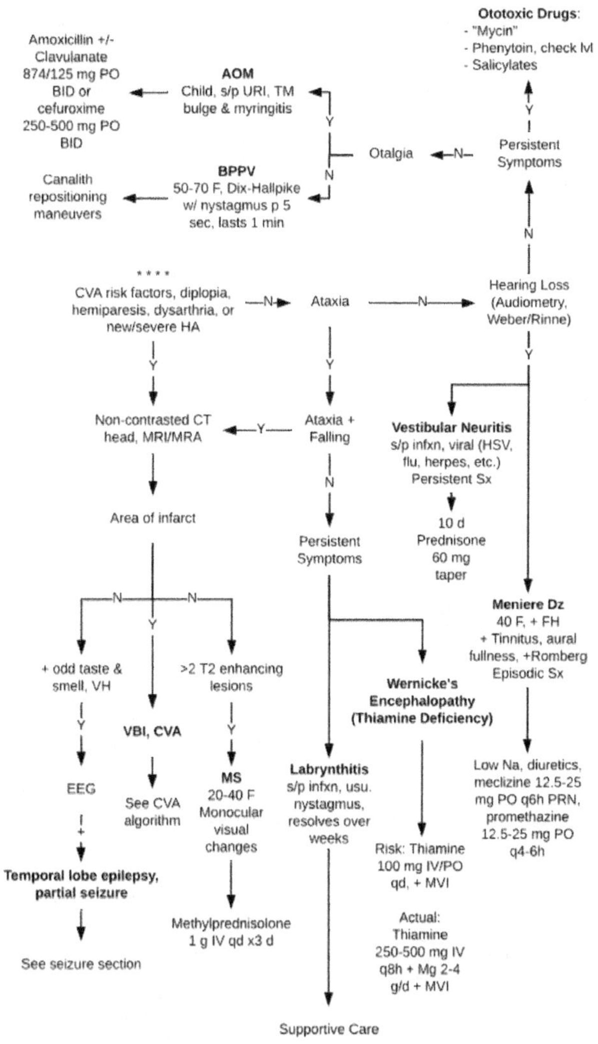
Ototoxic Drugs:
- "Mycin"
- Phenytoin, check lvl
- Salicylates
Amoxicillin +/- Clavulanate 874/125 mg PO BID or cefuroxime 250-500 mg PO BID
AOM
Child, s/p URI, TM bulge & myringitis
Y
Otalgia
N
Persistent Symptoms
BPPV
50-70 F, Dix-Hallpike w/ nystagmus p 5 sec, lasts 1 min
Canalith repositioning maneuvers
N
****
CVA risk factors, diplopia, hemiparesis, dysarthria, or new/severe HA
Ataxia
Hearing Loss (Audiometry, Weber/Rinne)
Y
Non-contrasted CT head, MRI/MRA
Ataxia + Falling
Vestibular Neuritis
s/p infxn, viral (HSV, flu, herpes, etc.)
Persistent Sx
10 d Prednisone 60 mg taper
Area of infarct
Persistent Symptoms
Meniere Dz
40 F, + FH
+ Tinnitus, aural fullness, +Romberg
Episodic Sx
+ odd taste & smell, VH
>2 T2 enhancing lesions
Wernicke's Encephalopathy (Thiamine Deficiency)
VBI, CVA
EEG
See CVA algorithm
MS
20-40 F
Monocular visual changes
Labrynthitis
s/p infxn, usu. nystagmus, resolves over weeks
Low Na, diuretics, meclizine 12.5-25 mg PO q6h PRN, promethazine 12.5-25 mg PO q4-6h
Risk: Thiamine 100 mg IV/PO qd, + MVI
Temporal lobe epilepsy, partial seizure
Methylprednisolone 1 g IV qd x3 d
Actual: Thiamine 250-500 mg IV q8h + Mg 2-4 g/d + MVI
See seizure section
Supportive Care

Weakness

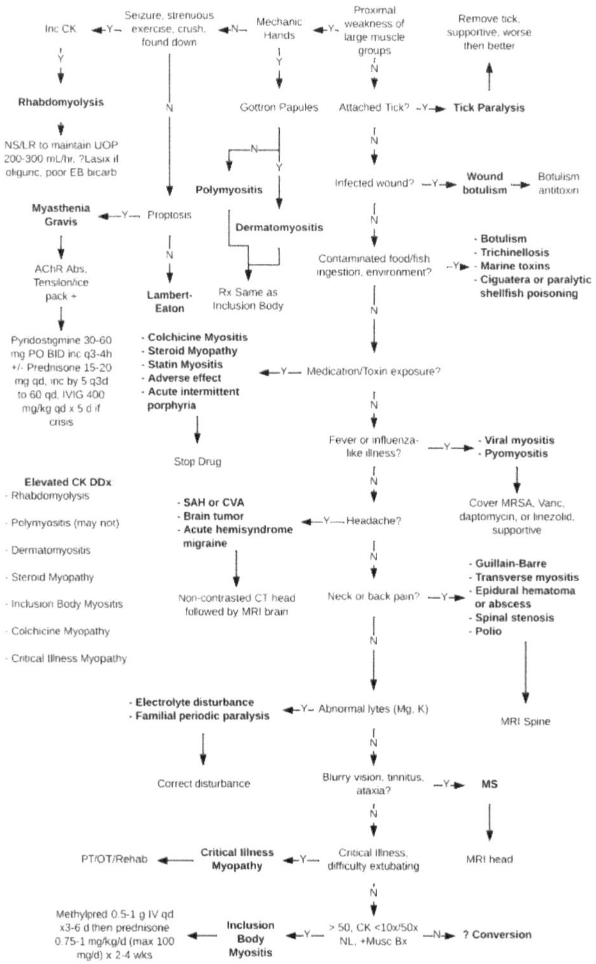
Inc CK
Seizure, strenuous exercise, crush, found down
Mechanic Hands
Proximal weakness of large muscle groups
Remove tick, supportive, worse then better
Y
N
Rhabdomyolysis
Gottron Papules
Attached Tick?
Tick Paralysis
NS/LR to maintain UOP 200-300 mL/hr, ?Lasix if oliguric, poor EB bicarb
Polymyositis
Infected wound?
Wound botulism
Botulism antitoxin
Myasthenia Gravis
Proptosis
Dermatomyositis
- Botulism
- Trichinellosis
- Marine toxins
- Ciguatera or paralytic shellfish poisoning
AChR Abs, Tensilon/ice pack +
Contaminated food/fish ingestion, environment?
Lambert-Eaton
Rx Same as Inclusion Body
Pyridostigmine 30-60 mg PO BID inc q3-4h +/- Prednisone 15-20 mg qd, inc by 5 q3d to 60 qd, IVIG 400 mg/kg qd x 5 d if crisis
- Colchicine Myositis
- Steroid Myopathy
- Statin Myositis
- Adverse effect
- Acute intermittent porphyria
Medication/Toxin exposure?
Stop Drug
Fever or influenza-like illness?
- Viral myositis
- Pyomyositis
Elevated CK DDx
- Rhabdomyolysis
- Polymyositis (may not)
- Dermatomyositis
- Steroid Myopathy
- Inclusion Body Myositis
- Colchicine Myopathy
- Critical Illness Myopathy
- SAH or CVA
- Brain tumor
- Acute hemisyndrome migraine
Headache?
Cover MRSA, Vanc, daptomycin, or linezolid, supportive
Non-contrasted CT head followed by MRI brain
Neck or back pain?
- Guillain-Barre
- Transverse myositis
- Epidural hematoma or abscess
- Spinal stenosis
- Polio
- Electrolyte disturbance
- Familial periodic paralysis
Abnormal lytes (Mg, K)
MRI Spine
Correct disturbance
Blurry vision, tinnitus, ataxia?
MS
PT/OT/Rehab
Critical Illness Myopathy
Critical Illness, difficulty extubating
MRI head
Methylpred 0.5-1 g IV qd x3-6 d then prednisone 0.75-1 mg/kg/d (max 100 mg/d) x 2-4 wks
Inclusion Body Myositis
> 50, CK <10x/50x NL, +Musc Bx
? Conversion

Tremor

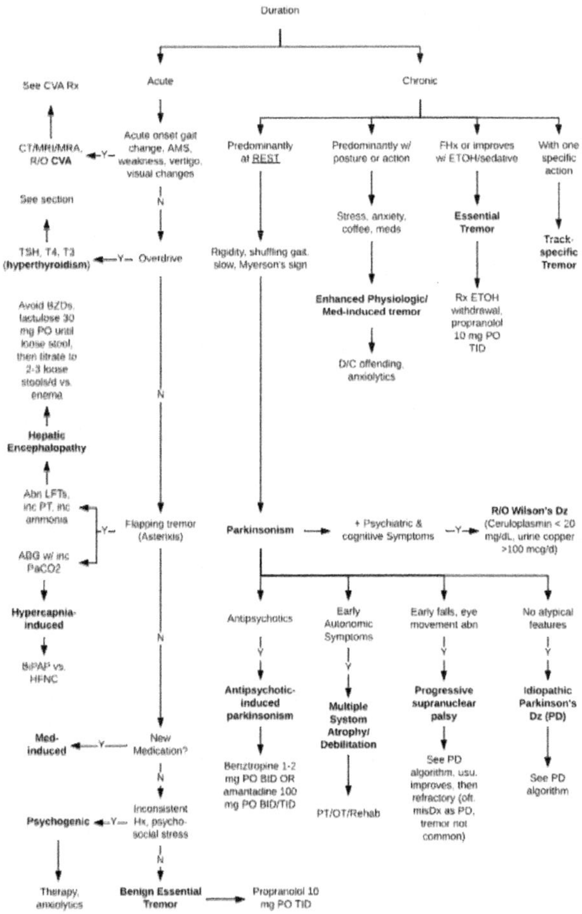
Duration
Acute
Chronic
See CVA Rx
CT/MRI/MRA, R/O CVA
Y
Acute onset gait change, AMS, weakness, vertigo, visual changes
N
See section
TSH, T4, T3 (hyperthyroidism)
Y
Overdrive
N
Avoid BZDs, lactulose 30 mg PO until loose stool, then titrate to 2-3 loose stools/d vs. enema
Hepatic Encephalopathy
Abn LFTs, inc PT, inc ammonia
Y
Flapping tremor (Asterixis)
ABG w/ inc PaCO2
Hypercapnia-induced
BiPAP vs. HFNC
N
Med-induced
Y
New Medication?
N
Psychogenic
Y
Inconsistent Hx, psycho-social stress
N
Therapy, anxiolytics
Benign Essential Tremor
Propranolol 10 mg PO TID
Predominantly at REST
Rigidity, shuffling gait, slow, Myerson's sign
Parkinsonism
+ Psychiatric & cognitive Symptoms
Y
R/O Wilson's Dz (Ceruloplasmin < 20 mg/dL, urine copper >100 mcg/d)
Predominantly w/ posture or action
Stress, anxiety, coffee, meds
Enhanced Physiologic/ Med-induced tremor
D/C offending, anxiolytics
FHx or improves w/ ETOH/sedative
Essential Tremor
Rx ETOH withdrawal, propranolol 10 mg PO TID
With one specific action
Track-specific Tremor
Antipsychotics
Y
Antipsychotic-induced parkinsonism
Benztropine 1-2 mg PO BID OR amantadine 100 mg PO BID/TID
Early Autonomic Symptoms
Y
Multiple System Atrophy/ Debilitation
PT/OT/Rehab
Early falls, eye movement abn
Y
Progressive supranuclear palsy
See PD algorithm, usu. improves, then refractory (oft. misDx as PD, tremor not common)
No atypical features
Y
Idiopathic Parkinson's Dz (PD)
See PD algorithm

Gait Abnormalities

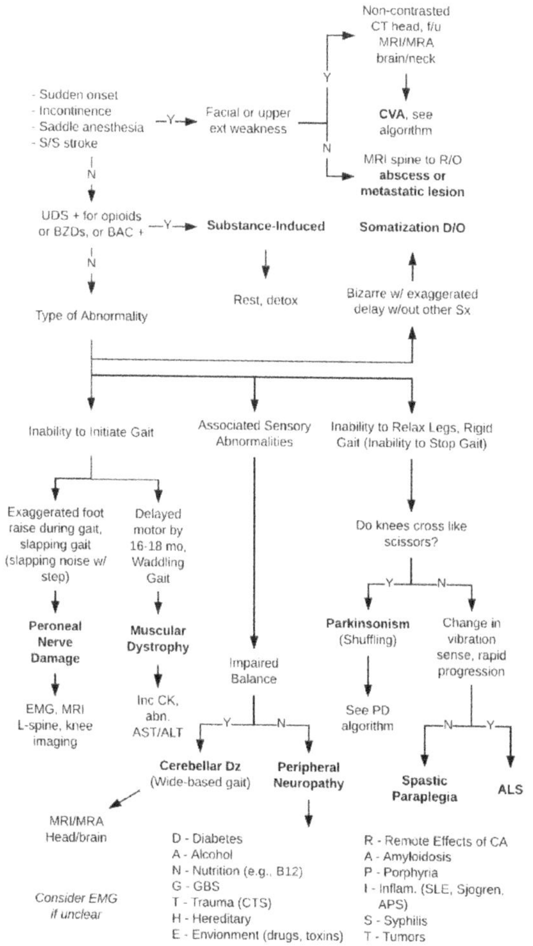

Urgent/Emergent Headache

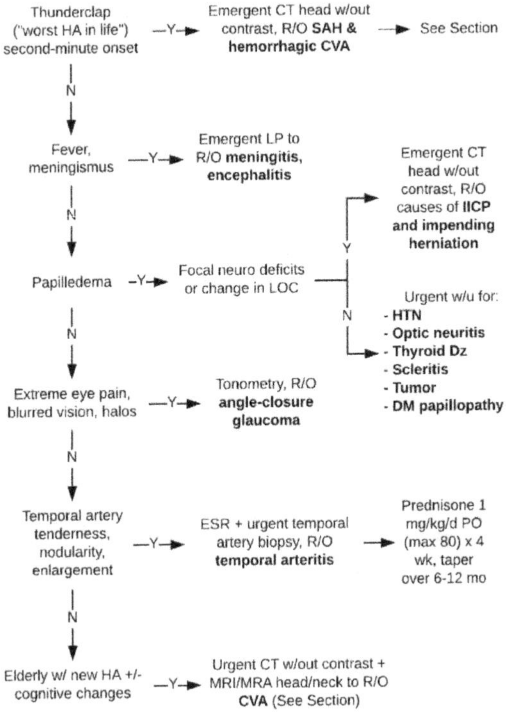

Secondary Headache

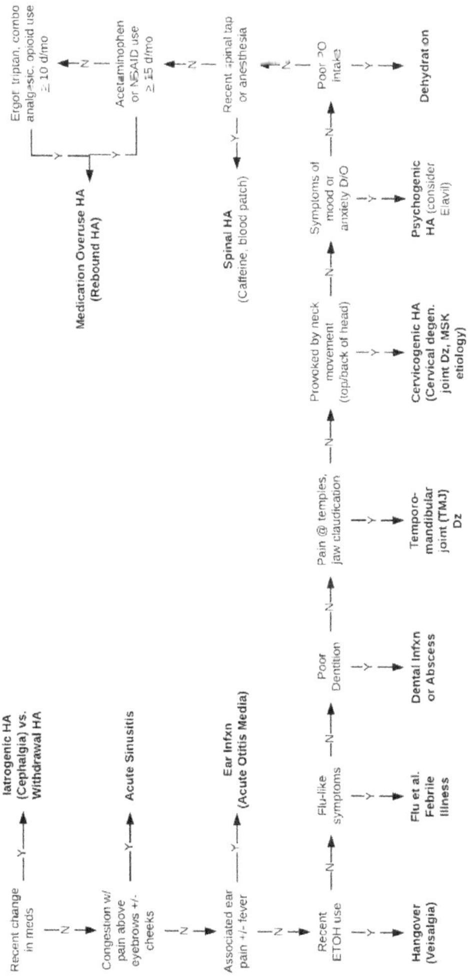

Primary Headache

P - Pulsating
O - hOurs (4-72)
U - Unilat
N - Nausea
D - Disabling
+/- Aura
Recurring "sinus" = migraine

—Y→ **Migraine**

↓ N

HA w/out nausea but ≥ 2:
- Bilat ("vise-like", tight)
- Non-pulsating pain
- Mild-mod pain
- Not provoked by activity

—Y→ **Tension-Type Headache**

↓ N

- Frequent HA
- Severe
- Brief (< 3 h per attack)
- Unilat (always same side)
- Ipsilat eye erythema, lacrimation, rhinorrhea, congestion
- Restlessness during attacks

—Y→ **Cluster HA et al. Trigeminal Autonomic Cephalgia (TAC)**

↓ N

- Unilateral
- Continuous
- Dramatically responsive to indomethacin

—Y→ **Hemicrania Continua**

↓ N

HA continuous since onset

—Y→ **New persistent daily HA**

Acute Headache Management

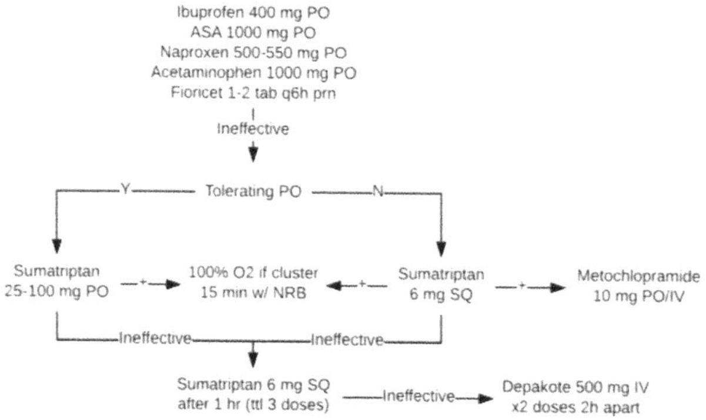

Prophylactic Headache Management

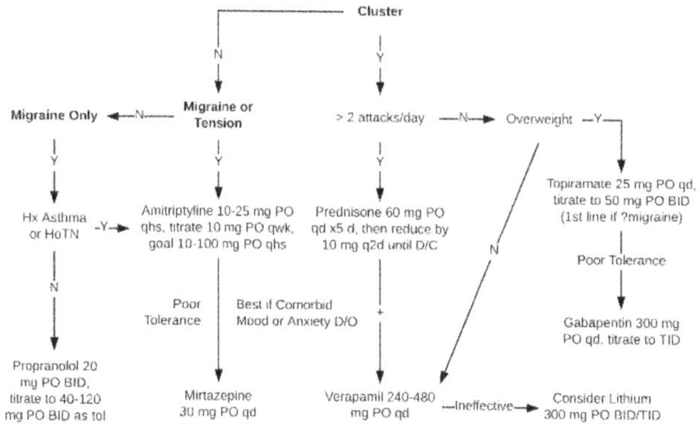

CVA and TIA

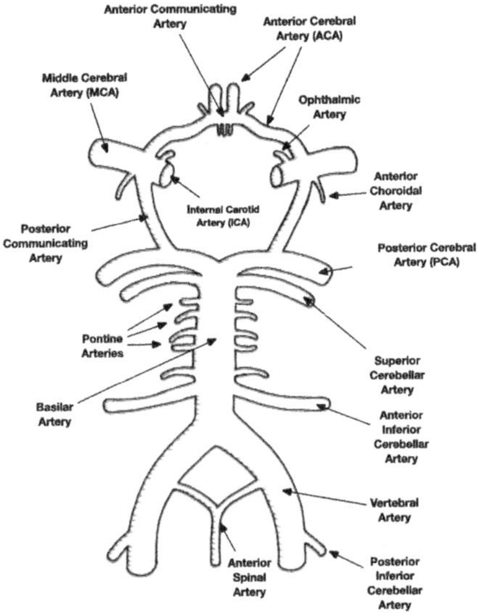

Artery	Effect & Notes
Middle Cerebral Artery (MCA)	Contralateral hemiparesis/hemiplegia, arm > leg
Anterior Branch	Language production (Broca's area) → Expressive aphasia
Posterior Branch	Language comprehension (Wernicke's area) → Receptive aphasia
Anterior Cerebral Artery (ACA)	Contralateral hemiparesis/hemiplegia, leg > arm; abulia or amotivation
Posterior Cerebral Artery (PCA)	Contralateral homonymous hemianopsia, CN III, contralateral hemiplegia
Basilar +/- Anterior Inferior Cerebellar Artery (AICA)	Pontine; ispilat CN V (face numb), CN VI (loss of abduction), CN VII (face weak), contralat. hemiplegia
Posterior Inferior Cerebellar Artery (PICA), Vertebral, +/- Basilar	Medullary; CN V (ipsilat face numb), CN VIII (vertigo, N/V), CN IX/X (dysarthria, dysphagia, uvula deviation away from lesion), CN XII (ipsilat tongue weakness, deviates toward lesion), Horner syndrome (ptosis, miosis), contralat hemiplegia/hemiparesis, ataxia
Posterior Circulation	Hemifield visual loss, cerebellar syndrome (ataxia); vertebrobasilar syndrome (HINTS exam, CTA or MRA)
Carotid Disease	Amaurosis fugax (transient loss of vision in 1-2 eyes) (Carotid US, CTA, or MRA)
Lacunar (small branches)	Isolated sensory/motor changes

"Non-specific white matter disease/microvascular disease" = risk of future CVA

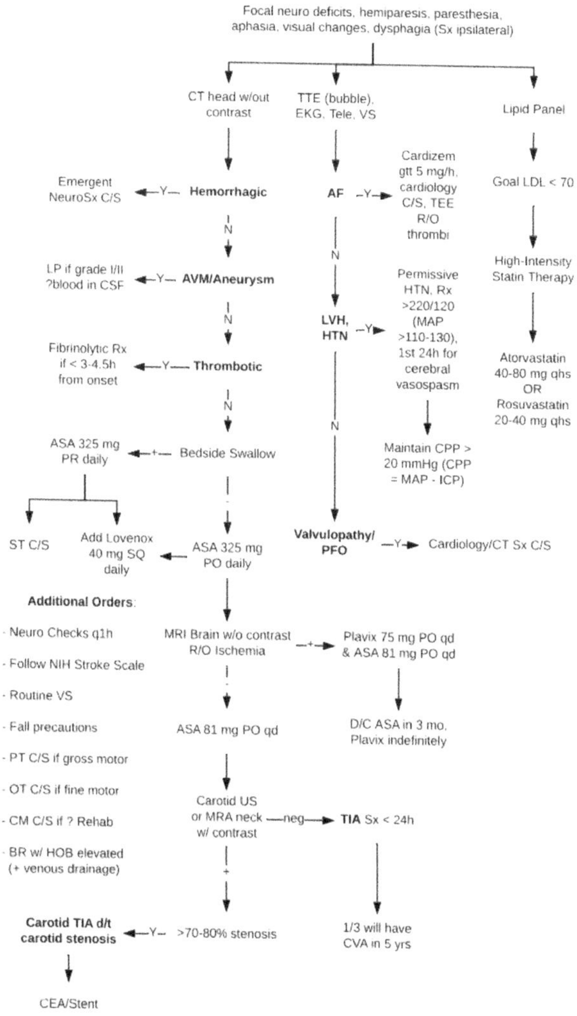
Focal neuro deficits, hemiparesis, paresthesia, aphasia, visual changes, dysphagia (Sx ipsilateral)
CT head w/out contrast
TTE (bubble), EKG, Tele, VS
Lipid Panel
Emergent NeuroSx C/S
Y
Hemorrhagic
N
AF
Y
Cardizem gtt 5 mg/h, cardiology C/S, TEE R/O thrombi
Goal LDL < 70
LP if grade I/II ?blood in CSF
Y
AVM/Aneurysm
N
N
Permissive HTN, Rx >220/120 (MAP >110-130), 1st 24h for cerebral vasospasm
High-Intensity Statin Therapy
LVH, HTN
Y
Fibrinolytic Rx if < 3-4.5h from onset
Y
Thrombotic
N
Atorvastatin 40-80 mg qhs OR Rosuvastatin 20-40 mg qhs
N
ASA 325 mg PR daily
+
Bedside Swallow
Maintain CPP > 20 mmHg (CPP = MAP - ICP)
-
ST C/S
Add Lovenox 40 mg SQ daily
ASA 325 mg PO daily
Valvulopathy/ PFO
Y
Cardiology/CT Sx C/S
Additional Orders:
- Neuro Checks q1h
- Follow NIH Stroke Scale
- Routine VS
- Fall precautions
- PT C/S if gross motor
- OT C/S if fine motor
- CM C/S if ? Rehab
- BR w/ HOB elevated (+ venous drainage)
MRI Brain w/o contrast R/O Ischemia
+
Plavix 75 mg PO qd & ASA 81 mg PO qd
-
ASA 81 mg PO qd
D/C ASA in 3 mo, Plavix indefinitely
Carotid US or MRA neck w/ contrast
neg
TIA Sx < 24h
+
Carotid TIA d/t carotid stenosis
Y
>70-80% stenosis
1/3 will have CVA in 5 yrs
CEA/Stent

Parkinson's Disease (PD)

A degenerative disorder d/t ↓ dopamine.

Epidemiology/Etiology:
- Occurs in all ethnic groups
- Approximately equal gender distribution
- Onset 45 – 65 y/o
- Most commonly idiopathic

Diagnosis:
- Clinical, no specific diagnostic

Manifestations:
- * Tremor: slow, esp. @ rest, pill rolling
- * Rigidity: resistant, cog wheel, jerky/slow
- * Bradykinesia: ↓ Blinking, dysphagia, drooling, poor movement initiation
    - ***Myerson's sign*** – repetitive tapping over bridge of nose → sustained blink
- * Postural instability: stooped, shuffling
- Mental deterioration +/- depression

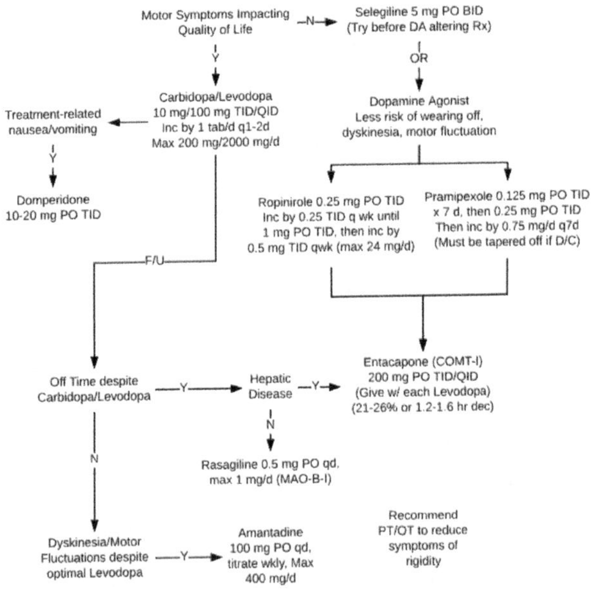

Ophthalmology

Visual Loss & Blurry Vision

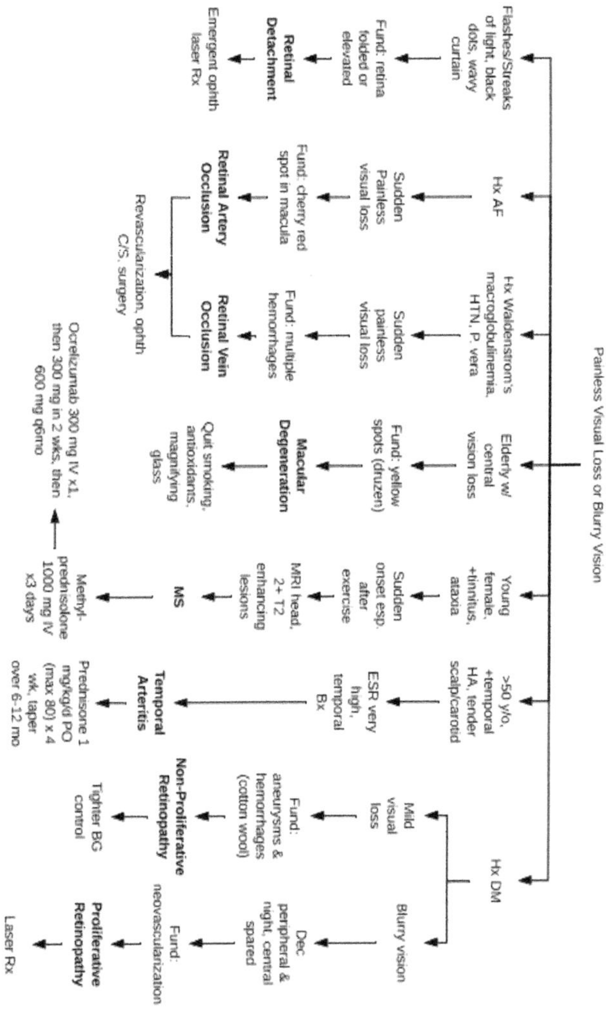

Red Eye, Severe Eye Pain

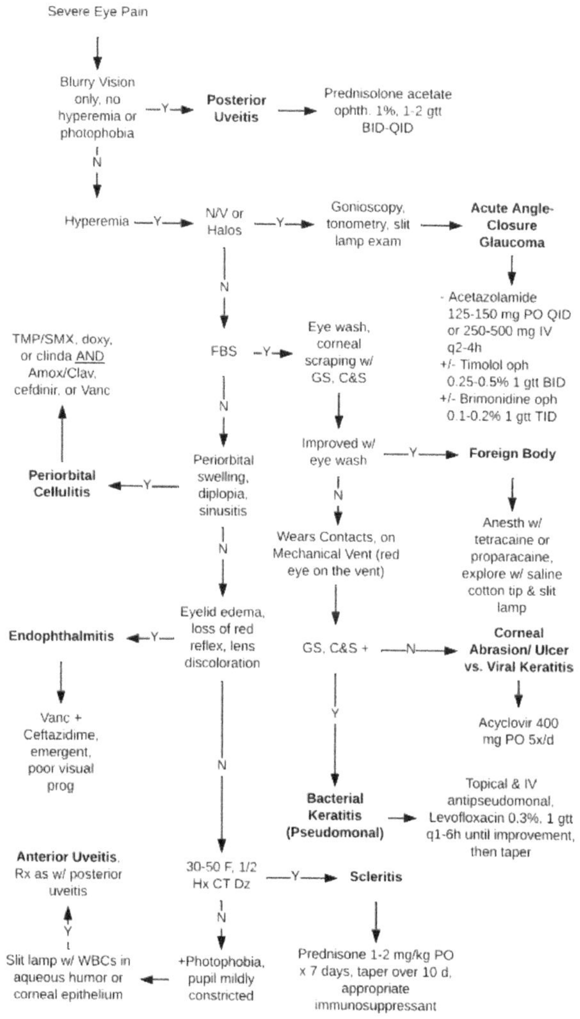

Red Eye, Without Severe Eye Pain

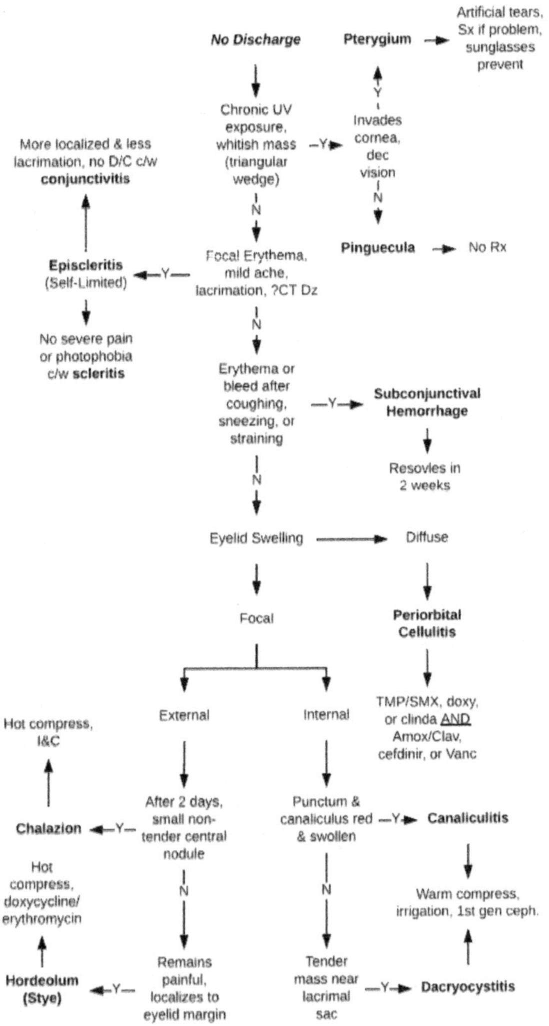

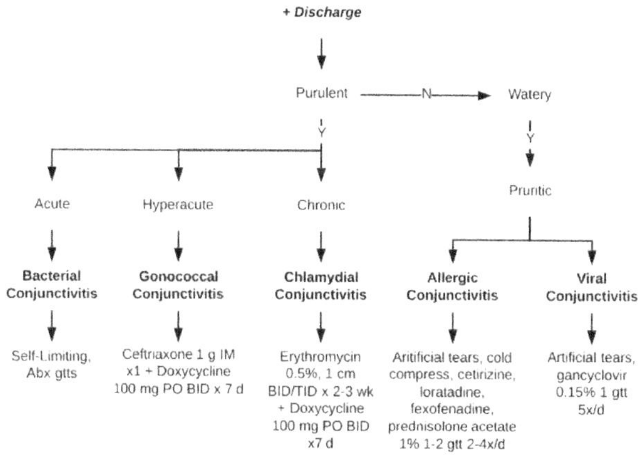

Lid Retraction or Proptosis

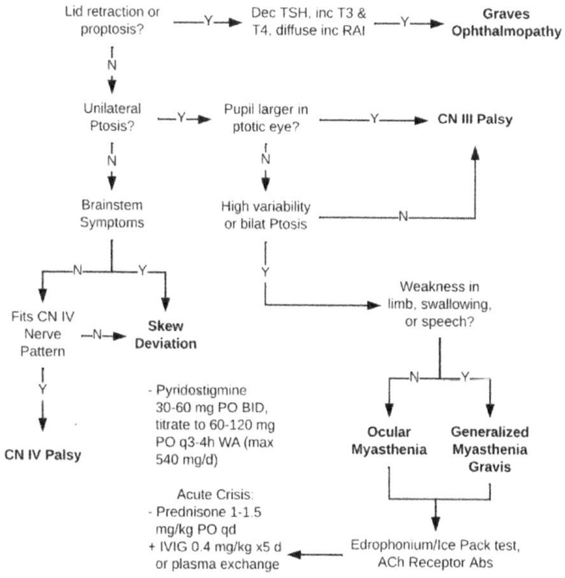

Diplopia

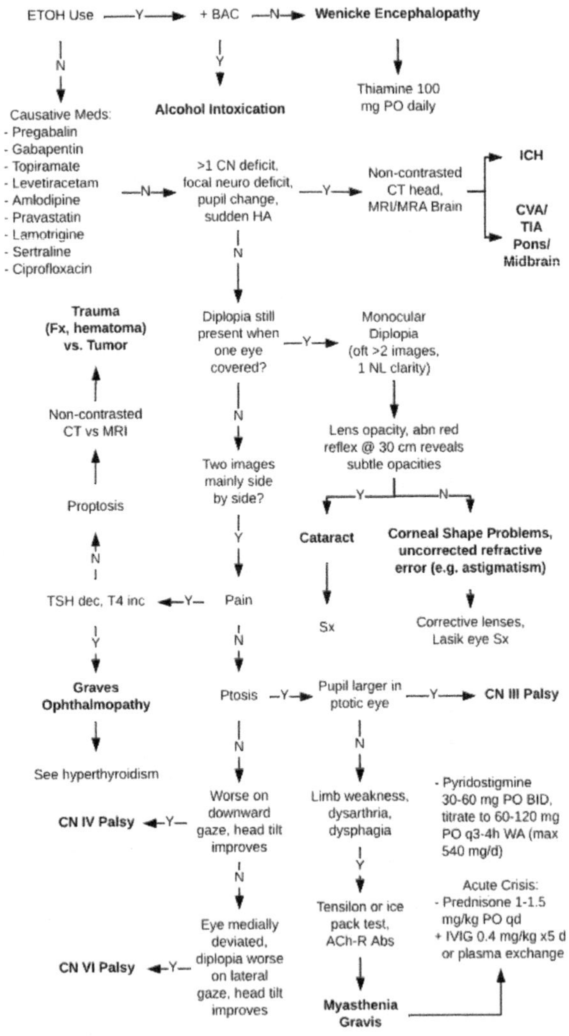
ETOH Use
Y
+ BAC
N
Wenicke Encephalopathy
N
Y
Thiamine 100 mg PO daily
Causative Meds:
- Pregabalin
- Gabapentin
- Topiramate
- Levetiracetam
- Amlodipine
- Pravastatin
- Lamotrigine
- Sertraline
- Ciprofloxacin
Alcohol Intoxication
N
>1 CN deficit, focal neuro deficit, pupil change, sudden HA
Y
Non-contrasted CT head, MRI/MRA Brain
ICH
CVA/ TIA Pons/ Midbrain
N
Trauma (Fx, hematoma) vs. Tumor
Diplopia still present when one eye covered?
Y
Monocular Diplopia (oft >2 images, 1 NL clarity)
Non-contrasted CT vs MRI
N
Lens opacity, abn red reflex @ 30 cm reveals subtle opacities
Two images mainly side by side?
Proptosis
Y
N
Cataract
Corneal Shape Problems, uncorrected refractive error (e.g. astigmatism)
N
Y
TSH dec, T4 inc
Y
Pain
Sx
Corrective lenses, Lasik eye Sx
Y
N
Graves Ophthalmopathy
Ptosis
Y
Pupil larger in ptotic eye
Y
CN III Palsy
See hyperthyroidism
N
N
- Pyridostigmine 30-60 mg PO BID, titrate to 60-120 mg PO q3-4h WA (max 540 mg/d)
CN IV Palsy
Y
Worse on downward gaze, head tilt improves
Limb weakness, dysarthria, dysphagia
N
Y
Acute Crisis:
- Prednisone 1-1.5 mg/kg PO qd
+ IVIG 0.4 mg/kg x5 d or plasma exchange
Tensilon or ice pack test, ACh-R Abs
CN VI Palsy
Y
Eye medially deviated, diplopia worse on lateral gaze, head tilt improves
Myasthenia Gravis

Otology

Acute Ear Pain

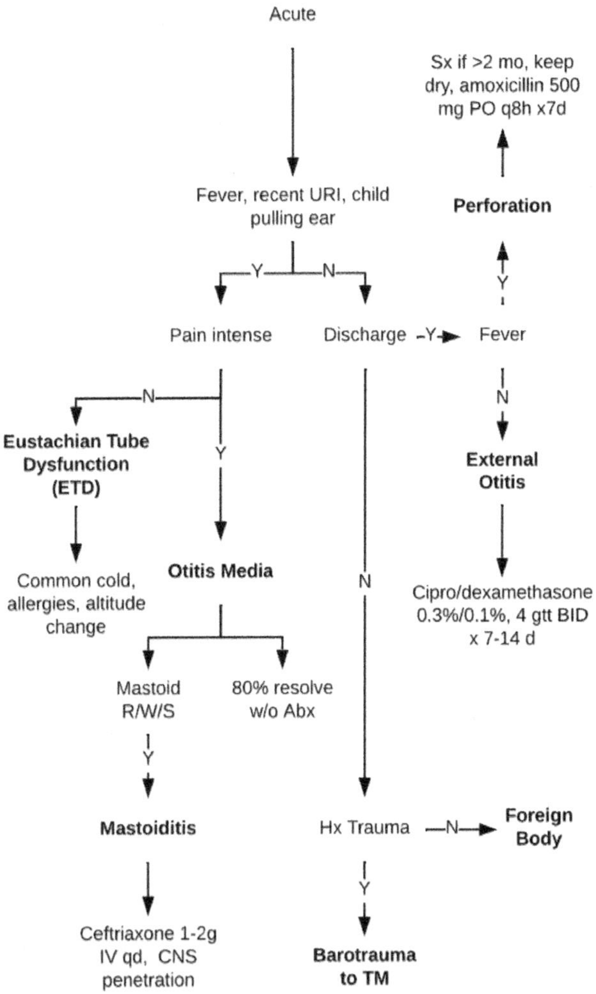

Chronic Ear Pain

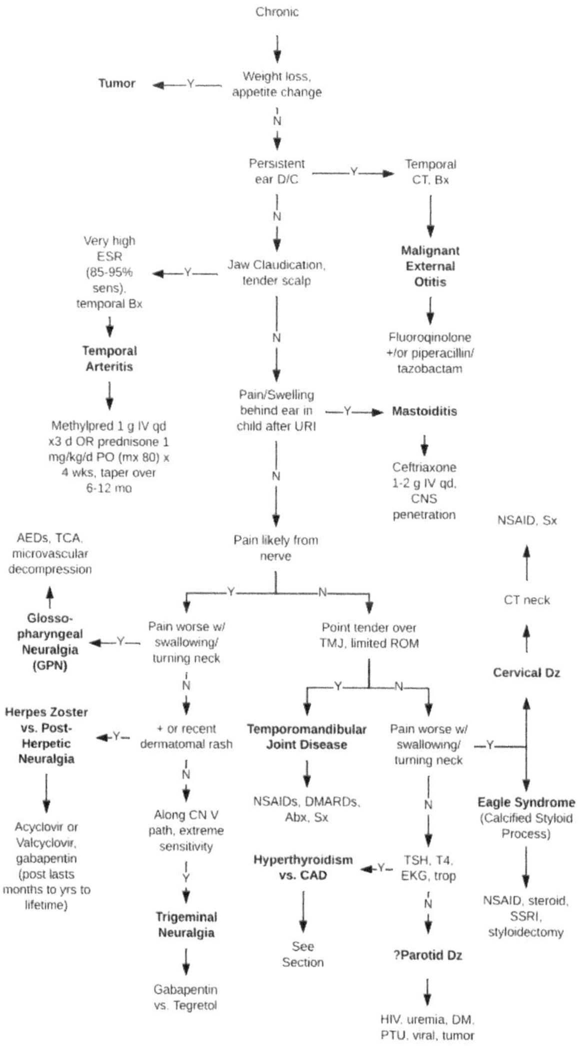

Tinnitus

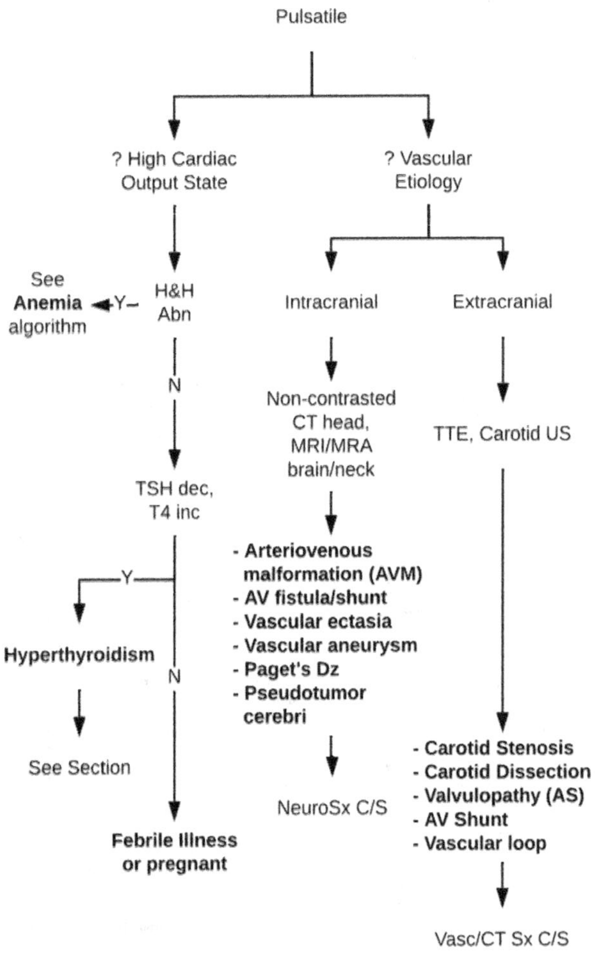
Pulsatile
? High Cardiac Output State
? Vascular Etiology
See **Anemia** algorithm
Y
H&H Abn
N
TSH dec, T4 inc
Y
Hyperthyroidism
See Section
N
Febrile Illness or pregnant
Intracranial
Non-contrasted CT head, MRI/MRA brain/neck
- **Arteriovenous malformation (AVM)**
- **AV fistula/shunt**
- **Vascular ectasia**
- **Vascular aneurysm**
- **Paget's Dz**
- **Pseudotumor cerebri**
NeuroSx C/S
Extracranial
TTE, Carotid US
- **Carotid Stenosis**
- **Carotid Dissection**
- **Valvulopathy (AS)**
- **AV Shunt**
- **Vascular loop**
Vasc/CT Sx C/S

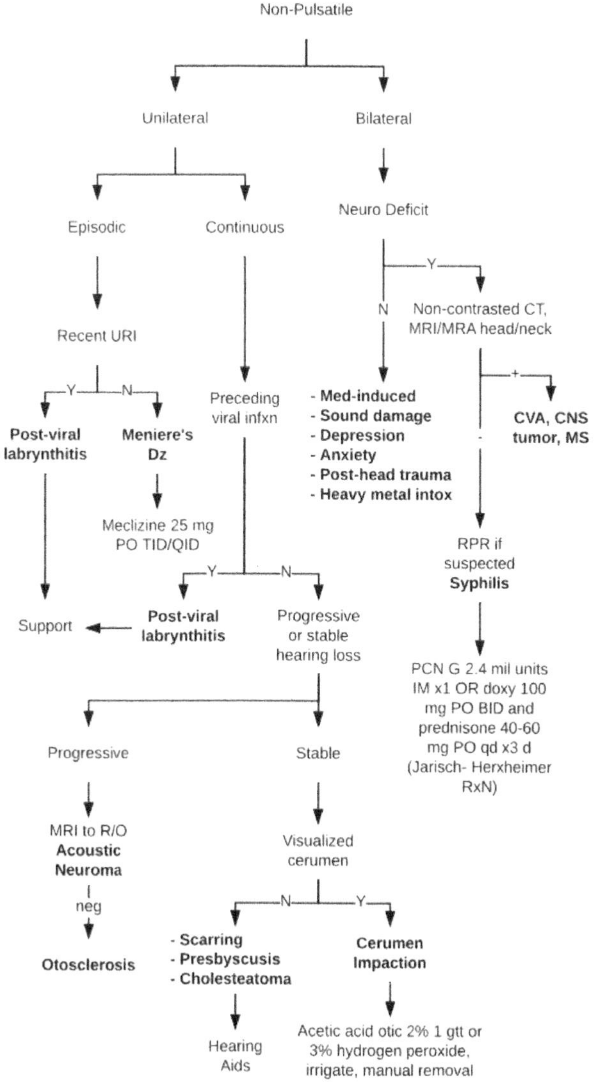
Non-Pulsatile
Unilateral
Bilateral
Episodic
Continuous
Neuro Deficit
Y
N
Non-contrasted CT, MRI/MRA head/neck
Recent URI
Y
N
Preceding viral infxn
- Med-induced
- Sound damage
- Depression
- Anxiety
- Post-head trauma
- Heavy metal intox
+
CVA, CNS tumor, MS
-
Post-viral labrynthitis
Meniere's Dz
Meclizine 25 mg PO TID/QID
RPR if suspected Syphilis
Y
N
Support
Post-viral labrynthitis
Progressive or stable hearing loss
PCN G 2.4 mil units IM x1 OR doxy 100 mg PO BID and prednisone 40-60 mg PO qd x3 d (Jarisch- Herxheimer RxN)
Progressive
Stable
MRI to R/O Acoustic Neuroma
neg
Visualized cerumen
N
Y
Otosclerosis
- Scarring
- Presbyscusis
- Cholesteatoma
Cerumen Impaction
Hearing Aids
Acetic acid otic 2% 1 gtt or 3% hydrogen peroxide, irrigate, manual removal

Hearing Loss

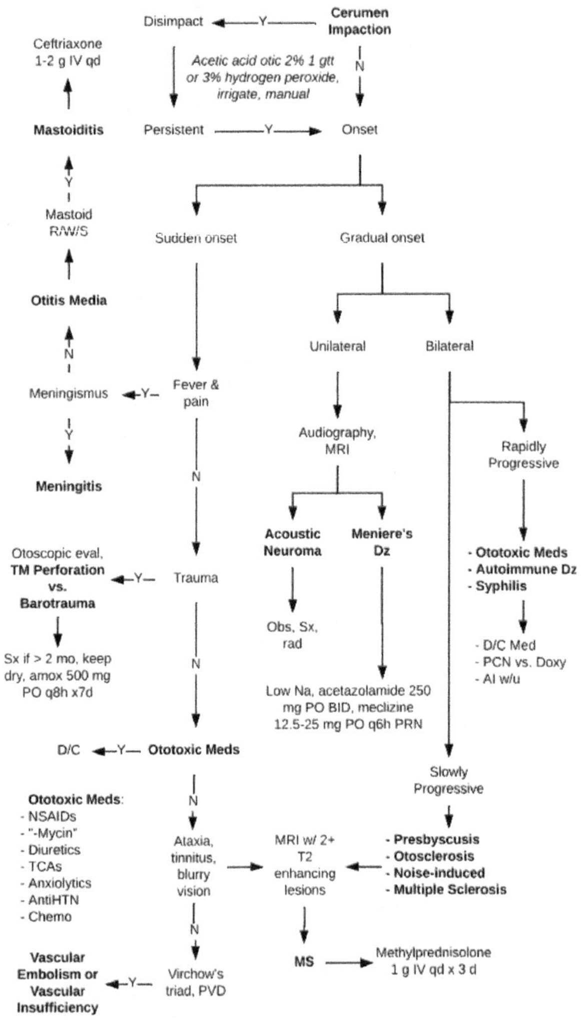

Pulmonology

Upper Respiratory Tract Infxn

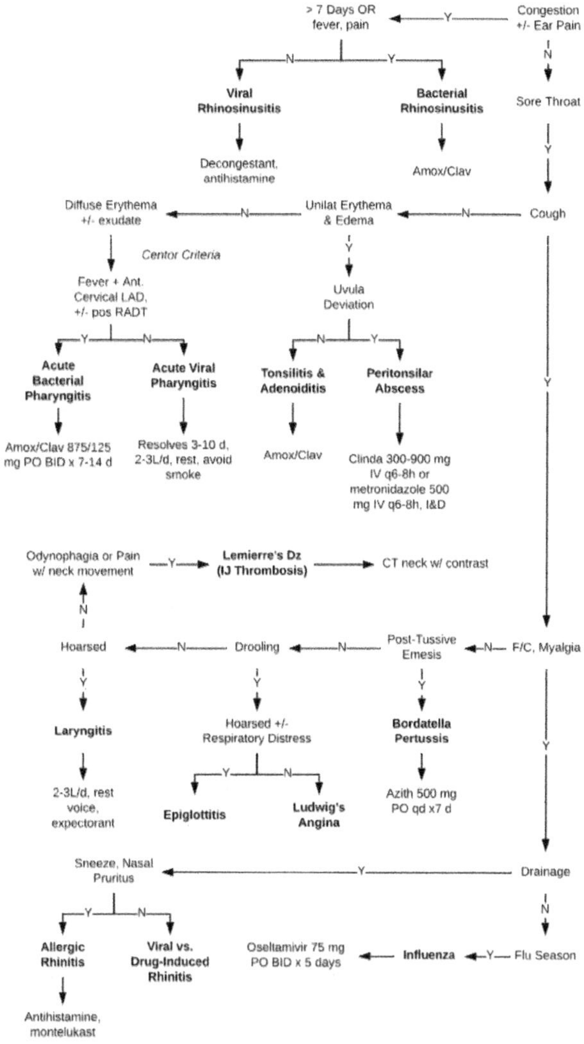

Acute Dyspnea

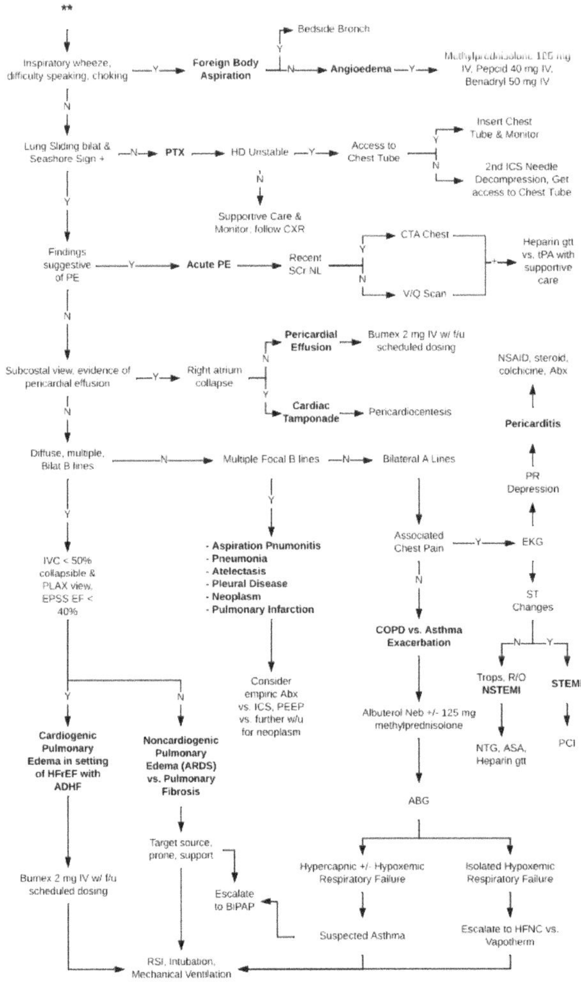

Cough

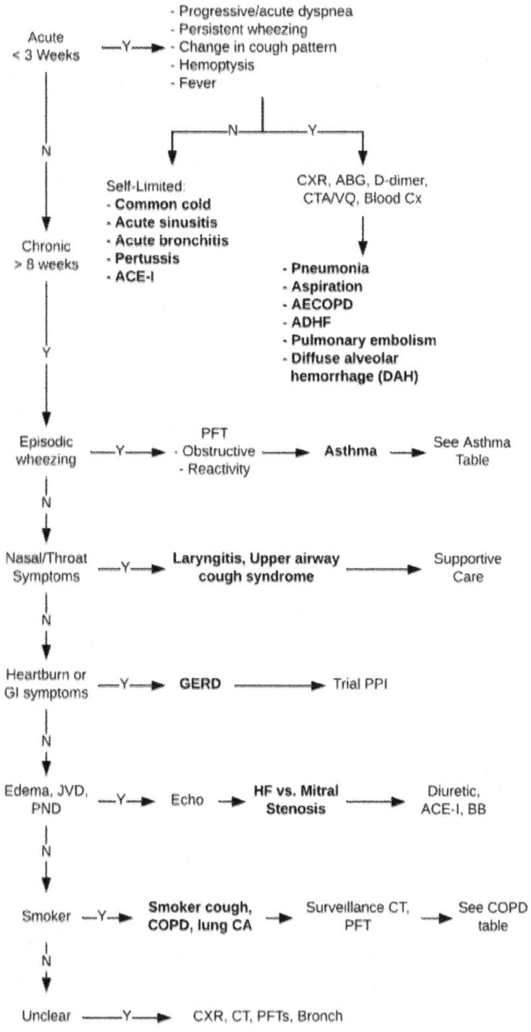

Acute
< 3 Weeks
Y
- Progressive/acute dyspnea
- Persistent wheezing
- Change in cough pattern
- Hemoptysis
- Fever
N
Y
Self-Limited:
- Common cold
- Acute sinusitis
- Acute bronchitis
- Pertussis
- ACE-I
CXR, ABG, D-dimer, CTA/VQ, Blood Cx
- Pneumonia
- Aspiration
- AECOPD
- ADHF
- Pulmonary embolism
- Diffuse alveolar hemorrhage (DAH)
N
Chronic
> 8 weeks
Y
Episodic wheezing
Y
PFT
- Obstructive
- Reactivity
Asthma
See Asthma Table
N
Nasal/Throat Symptoms
Y
Laryngitis, Upper airway cough syndrome
Supportive Care
N
Heartburn or GI symptoms
Y
GERD
Trial PPI
N
Edema, JVD, PND
Y
Echo
HF vs. Mitral Stenosis
Diuretic, ACE-I, BB
N
Smoker
Y
Smoker cough, COPD, lung CA
Surveillance CT, PFT
See COPD table
N
Unclear
Y
CXR, CT, PFTs, Bronch

Hemoptysis

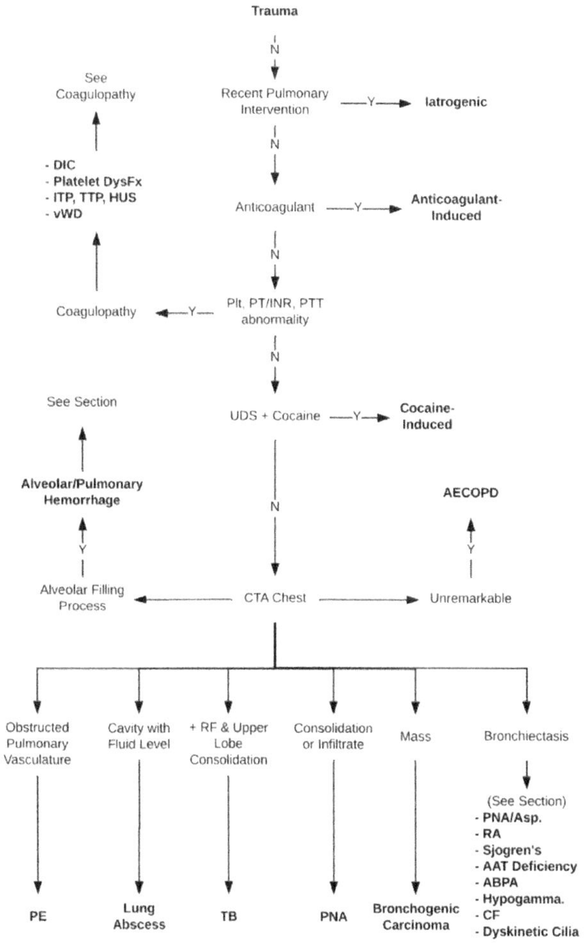

Inhaled Tranexamic Acid 500 mg TID, safe & effective in non-massive hemoptysis (Wand et al., 2018)

Hypoxemia

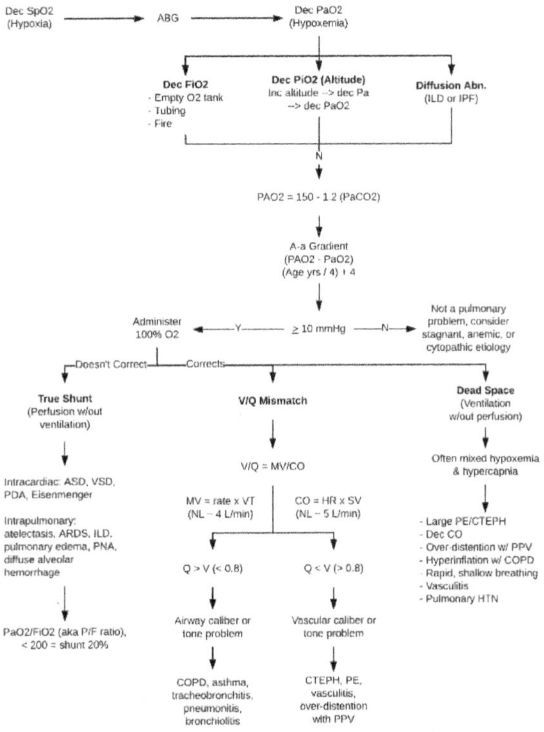

Four Types of Hypoxemia

Hypoxemic – low PaO_2/SaO_2 leading to low delivery of O_2 to the tissues

Stagnant – low cardiac output, which leads to tissue hypoxia even if the pt is breathing 100% oxygen

Anemic – not enough red blood cells to carry oxygen to the tissues

Cytopathic – the heart pumps enough oxygen to the tissues, but something inhibits effective oxidative phosphorylation (e.g., septic shock, cyanide poisoning, salicylate poisoning)

More Hypoxemia Analysis

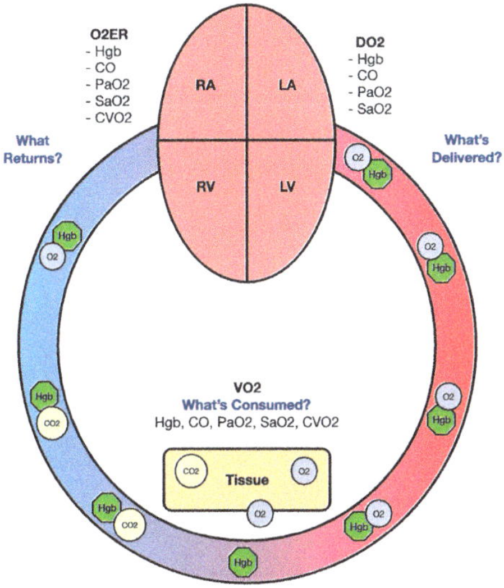

Oxygen Content

$CaO_2 = 1.34\ (Hgb)\ (SaO_2) + 0.003\ (PaO_2)$, NL ~ 20 mL O_2/dL blood

Oxygen Delivery

What's delivered to the toes?

$DO_2 = CaO_2 \times CO \times 10$

NL ~ 1,000 mL O_2/min

Oxygen Consumption

What's used at the cellular level?

$VO_2 = (CaO_2 - C_VO_2) \times CO \times 10$

NL ~ 250 mL O_2/min

Oxygen Extraction Ratio

After determining what was delivered and what was consumed... what's left?

$O_2ER = VO_2/DO_2$

Alternatively: $O_2ER = (SaO_2 - S_VO_2) / (SaO_2)$

NL ~ 25%

Hypoxemic Respiratory Failure if PaO2 < 60 mmHg

Hypercapnic/Hypercarbic Respiratory Failure if PaCO2 >50 mmHg

The Oxyhemoglobin Dissociation Curve

Relationship between SaO2 & PaO2. The higher the PaO2, the more readily O2 combines w/ Hgb (HbO2)

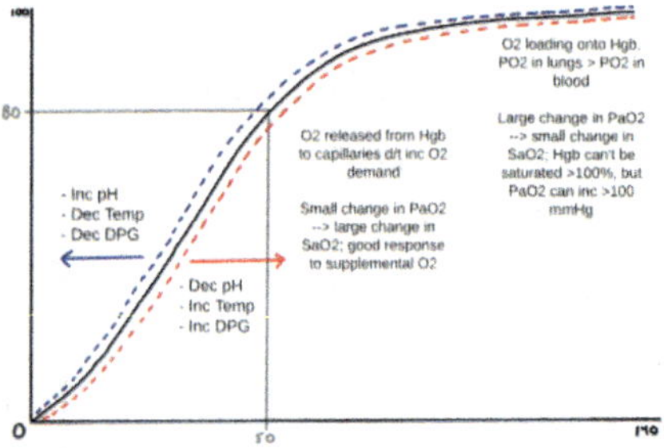

Curve to Right: O_2 affinity for Hgb ↓ (O_2 becomes more available to tissues

Curve to Left: O_2 affinity for Hgb ↑ (reduces availability of O_2 to tissues)

Bohr effect – OHDC shifts to right in systemic circulation facilitating unloading of O_2 from blood to tissues; shifts to left in pulmonary circulation facilitating loading of O_2

Hypoventilation & Hypercapnia

Can produce hypoxemia (often easily reversible with O_2), but most often produces hypercapnia. Think about where the problem is!

Brainstem:

- Drug OD
- Trauma
- ICH/SAH
- Infxn
- OHS
- Hepatic/uremic encephalopathy

Spinal Cord:

- Lesion C4 or higher
- Traumatic brain injury (TBI)
- Spinal anesthesia
- Epidural abscess

Peripheral Nerves:

- Phrenic nerve paralysis
- Tick paralysis
- GBS
- Heavy metal poisoning

Neuromuscular Junction (NMJ):

- Botulism
- MG
- NMBs

Muscles:

- Muscular dystrophy (MD)
- Hypothyroidism
- Hypokalemia
- Hypophosphatemia
- Hypomagnesemia

Thoracic Cage:

- Kyphoscoliosis
- Morbid obesity (OHS)
- Flail chest
- Ankylosing spondylitis

Lungs: COPD, etc.

Pulmonary Function Testing (PFT)

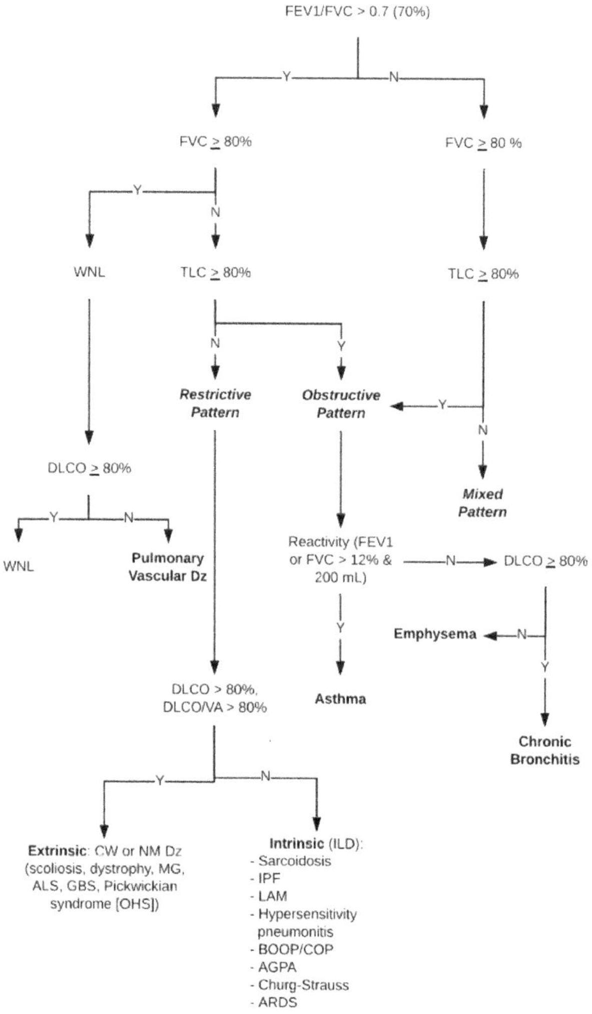

Flow Volume Loop

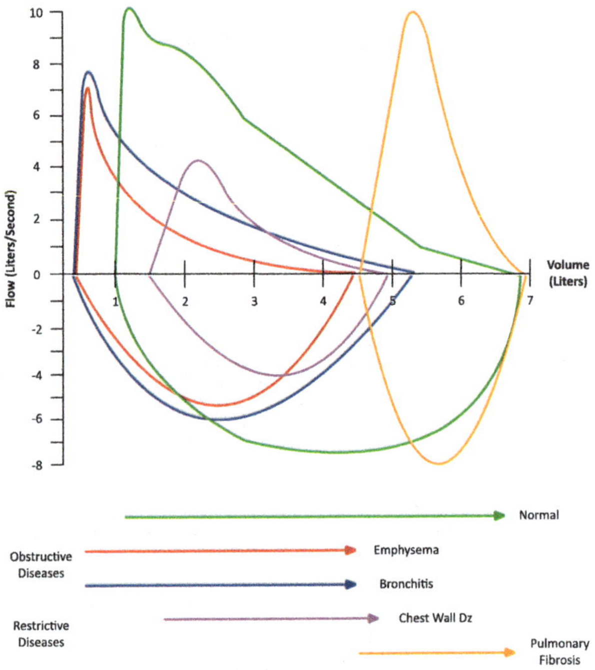

Chest X-ray

CLAVICLE Mnemonic

C – Correct Patient and Film

L – Life Support Devices

A – Anatomy

V – Vascular Structures

I – Interfaces

C – Categorize the Parenchymal Pattern

L – Limitations

E – Extra Look

Pattern Approach

1. **Consolidation**: alveoli filled with fluid, pus, blood, cells.
   - Multiple ill-defined pattern
   - Lobar pattern
   - Diffuse pattern
   - Batwing & reversed batwing

2. **Atelectasis**: collapse d/t ↓ air in alveoli → volume loss & ↑ density

3. **Nodule or mass**: space-occupying lesion.
   - Solitary pulmonary nodule
   - Multiple masses

4. **Interstitial**: lung parenchyma process.
   - Fine or coarse reticular opacities
   - Nodular interstitial opacities

5. ↓ **density/Lucencies**: cavity, cyst, multiple

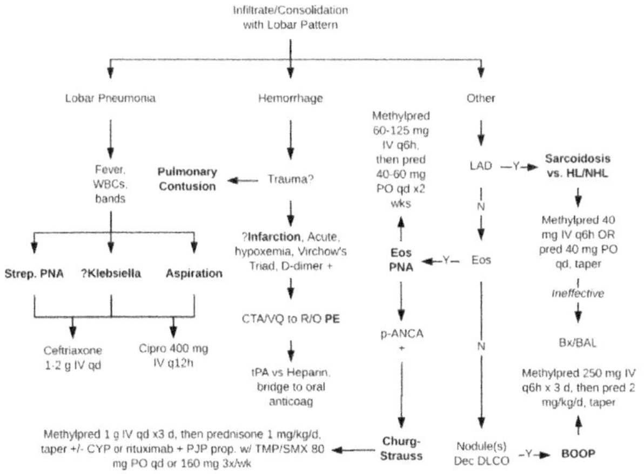

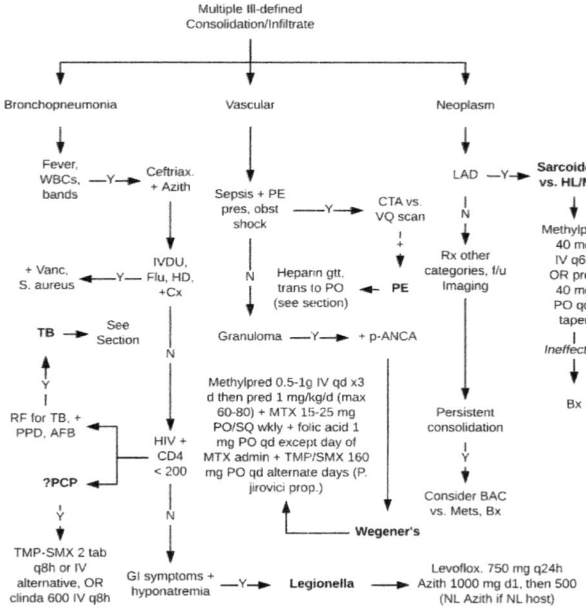
Multiple Ill-defined Consolidation/Infiltrate
Bronchopneumonia
Vascular
Neoplasm
Fever, WBCs, bands
Y
Ceftriax. + Azith
IVDU, Flu, HD, +Cx
Y
+ Vanc, S. aureus
N
HIV + CD4 < 200
RF for TB, + PPD, AFB
Y
TB
See Section
?PCP
Y
TMP-SMX 2 tab q8h or IV alternative, OR clinda 600 IV q8h
N
GI symptoms + hyponatremia
Y
Legionella
Levoflox. 750 mg q24h Azith 1000 mg d1, then 500 (NL Azith if NL host)
Sepsis + PE pres, obst shock
Y
CTA vs. VQ scan
+
PE
Heparin gtt, trans to PO (see section)
N
Granuloma
Y
+ p-ANCA
Wegener's
Methylpred 0.5-1g IV qd x3 d then pred 1 mg/kg/d (max 60-80) + MTX 15-25 mg PO/SQ wkly + folic acid 1 mg PO qd except day of MTX admin + TMP/SMX 160 mg PO qd alternate days (P. jirovici prop.)
LAD
Y
Sarcoidosis vs. HL/NHL
Methylpred 40 mg IV q6h OR pred 40 mg PO qd, taper
Ineffective
Bx
N
Rx other categories, f/u Imaging
Persistent consolidation
Y
Consider BAC vs. Mets, Bx

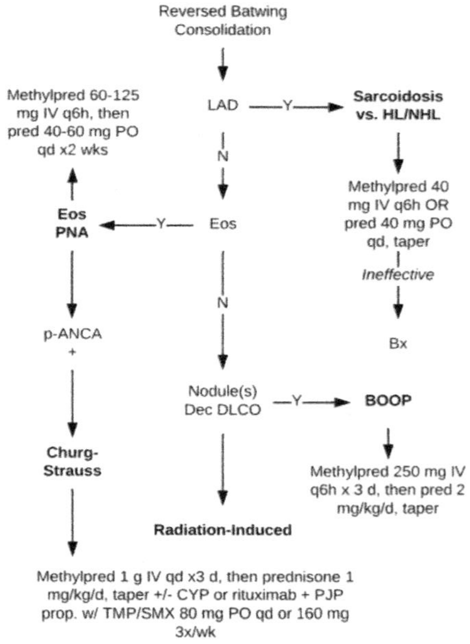
Reversed Batwing Consolidation
LAD
Y
Sarcoidosis vs. HL/NHL
Methylpred 40 mg IV q6h OR pred 40 mg PO qd, taper
Ineffective
Bx
N
Eos
Y
Eos PNA
Methylpred 60-125 mg IV q6h, then pred 40-60 mg PO qd x2 wks
p-ANCA +
Churg-Strauss
Methylpred 1 g IV qd x3 d, then prednisone 1 mg/kg/d, taper +/- CYP or rituximab + PJP prop. w/ TMP/SMX 80 mg PO qd or 160 mg 3x/wk
N
Nodule(s) Dec DLCO
Y
BOOP
Methylpred 250 mg IV q6h x 3 d, then pred 2 mg/kg/d, taper
Radiation-Induced

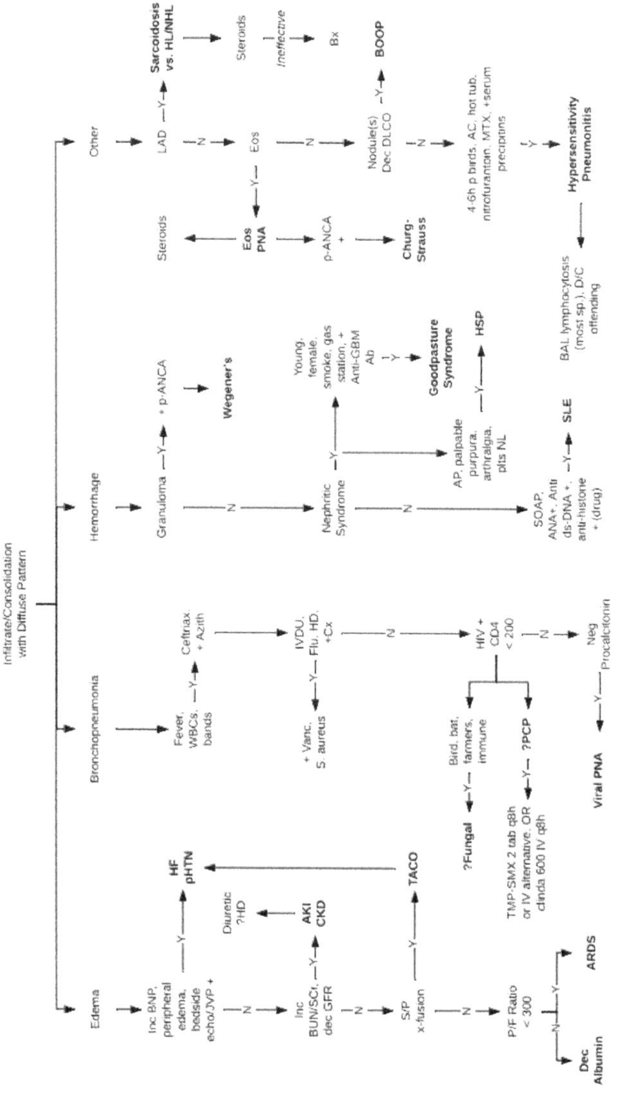
Infiltrate/Consolidation with Diffuse Pattern
Edema
Bronchopneumonia
Hemorrhage
Other
Inc BNP, peripheral edema, bedside echo/JVP +
HF pHTN
Diuretic ?HD
Inc BUN/SCr, dec GFR
AKI CKD
S/P x-fusion
TACO
P/F Ratio < 300
ARDS
Dec Albumin
Fever, WBCs, bands
Ceftriax + Azith
IVDU, Flu, HD, +Cx
+ Vanc, S. aureus
HIV + CD4 < 200
Bird, bat, farmers, immune
?Fungal
?PCP
TMP-SMX 2 tab q8h or IV alternative, OR clinda 600 IV q8h
Neg Procalcitonin
Viral PNA
Granuloma
+ p-ANCA
Wegener's
Nephritic Syndrome
Young, female, smoke, gas station, + Anti-GBM Ab
Goodpasture Syndrome
AP, palpable purpura, arthralgia, plts NL
HSP
SOAP, ANA+, Anti ds-DNA +, anti-histone + (drug)
SLE
LAD
Sarcoidosis vs. HL/NHL
Steroids
Ineffective
Bx
Eos
Eos PNA
p-ANCA +
Churg-Strauss
Nodule(s) Dec DLCO
BOOP
4-6h p birds, AC, hot tub, nitrofurantoin, MTX, +serum precipitins
Hypersensitivity Pneumonitis
BAL lymphocytosis (most sp.), D/C offending
Y
N

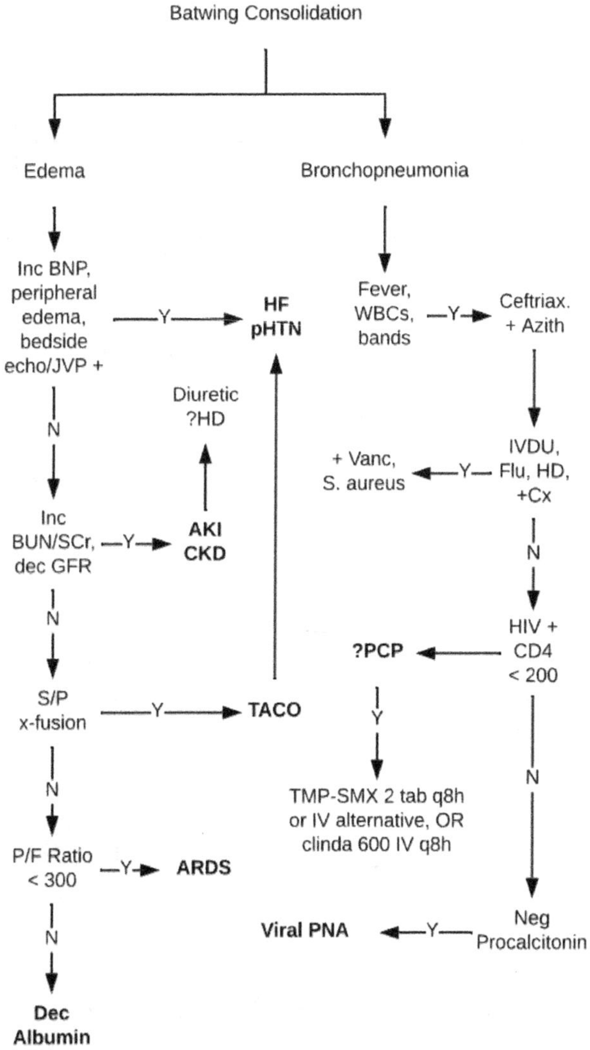
Batwing Consolidation
Edema
Bronchopneumonia
Inc BNP, peripheral edema, bedside echo/JVP +
Y
HF
pHTN
Fever, WBCs, bands
Y
Ceftriax. + Azith
N
Diuretic ?HD
IVDU, Flu, HD, +Cx
Y
+ Vanc, S. aureus
Inc BUN/SCr, dec GFR
Y
AKI
CKD
N
N
HIV + CD4 < 200
?PCP
S/P x-fusion
Y
TACO
Y
N
TMP-SMX 2 tab q8h or IV alternative, OR clinda 600 IV q8h
N
P/F Ratio < 300
Y
ARDS
N
Neg Procalcitonin
Y
Viral PNA
Dec Albumin

Atelectasis

Key Findings on CXR: Sharply defined opacity obscuring vessels w/out air bronchogram, volume loss resulting in displacement of diaphragm fissures, hili, or mediastinum (e.g., diaphragmatic tenting)

Reabsorption	Relaxation
- Mucus plugging (mechanical vent, ABPA) - Tumor (bronchial carcinoma) - Foreign body	- Pleural effusion - Pneumothorax - Rounded atelectasis (pleural-based mass or pleuritis)

Multiple Masses DDx

Neoplastic	Inflammatory
- Metastases (renal, GI, melanoma, uterus, testis, sarcoma) - Uncommon: bronchoalveolar cell cancer, lymphoma, Kaposi	- Sarcoidosis - RA-nodules - Wegener's granulomas - Organizing pneumonia
Infection	**Vascular**
- TB - Fungal (histoplasmosis, coccidiomycosis, invasive aspergillosis) - Septic emboli	- Osler-Weber-Rendu (AVM) - Pulmonary infarcts **Inhalation** - Mucoid impaction (ABPA) - Silicosis

↓ Density or Lucencies

Cavity (wall > 3 mm)	Cyst (wall ≤ 3 mm)
Infxn: - Staphylococcus/Klebsiella - Gram negative organism - Anaerobe in aspiration - TB, fungal (aspergillus) Neoplasm: Lung CA (SCLC, BAC), Metastases Vascular: Lung infarction	Congenital: - Bronchogenic cyst - Cystic adenomatoid malformation (CAM) Bulla Pneumatocele: - Post-traumatic

Multiple		
Infxn: - Staphylococcus/Klebsiella - Gram negative organism - Anaerobe in aspiration - TB, fungal (e.g., aspergillus), PCP	Neoplasm: - Lung CA (SCLC, BAC) - Metastases Collagen-vascular: - Thrombo-/septic emboli - RA, Wegener's	Emphysema Cystic Lung Dz: - PLCH - Lymphangio-leiomyomatosis - Honeycombing

Radiological Patterns on CT

Ground Glass & Consolidation	Fibrosis

- Edema
- Infection
- Aspiration
- Hypersensitivity pneumonitis
- Drug reactions
- Fumes and toxin injury
- Related to rheumatic disease
- Idiopathic interstitial pneumonias
    - Non-specific interstitial PNA (NSIP)
    - Lymphocytic interstitial PNA (LIP)
    - Desquamative interstitial PNA
- Bronchiolitis-associated ILD
- Lymphangitic tumors
- Wegener granulomatosis
- Alveolar proteinosis
- Amyloidosis
	- Pneumoconiosis
	- Chronic granulomatous infxn
	- Usual interstitial pneumonia (UIP)
	- Chronic hypersensitivity pneumonitis
	- Related to rheumatic disease
	- Chronic drug reactions
	- Sarcoidosis
	- Lymphocytic interstitial PNA (LIP)
	- Chronic aspiration
	- Chronic radiation injury
	- Advanced Pulmonary Langerhans Cell histiocytosis (PLCH)
	- Hermansky-Pudlak syndrome
	- Erdheim-Chester Dz (non Langerhans cell histiocytosis)

Nodules	**Mosaic Pattern/Cysts**
- Carcinomas and sarcomas - Lymphoproliferative Dzs - Military granulomatous infxns - Aspiration bronchiolitis - Hypersensitivity pneumonitis - Pulmonary Langerhans cell Histiocytosis (PLCH) - Sarcoidosis - Wegener granulomatosis - Necrotizing sarcoidosis - Silicosis and silicate Dz	- Small-airways Dz with constrictive bronchiolitis - Vasculopathic diseases - Lymphangioleiomyomatosis - Pulmonary Langerhans cell histiocytosis (PLCH)

Solitary Pulmonary Nodule

Most Common	Uncommon/Rare
- Granuloma **Less Common** - Bronchial carcinoma - Metastasis - Organizing pneumonia - Hamartoma	- Mucoid impaction - Abscess - Infected bulla - Infarction - Hematoma - Rheumatoid nodule - Wegener's granuloma - Carcinoid - Sarcoid granuloma - Arteriovenous malformation - Intrapulmonary lipoma or lymph node - Hydatid cyst

Pulmonary Nodule

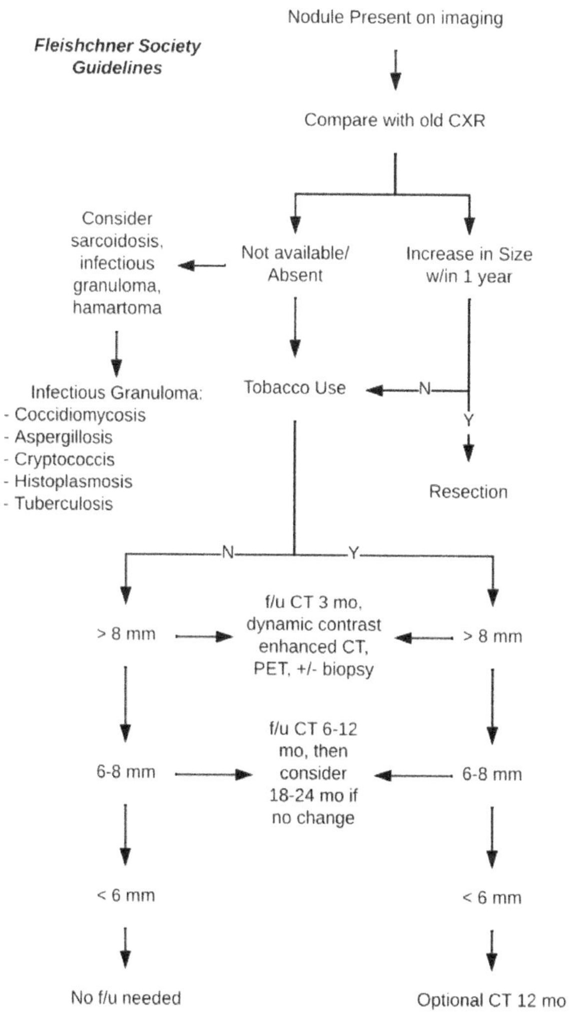

Bronchiectasis

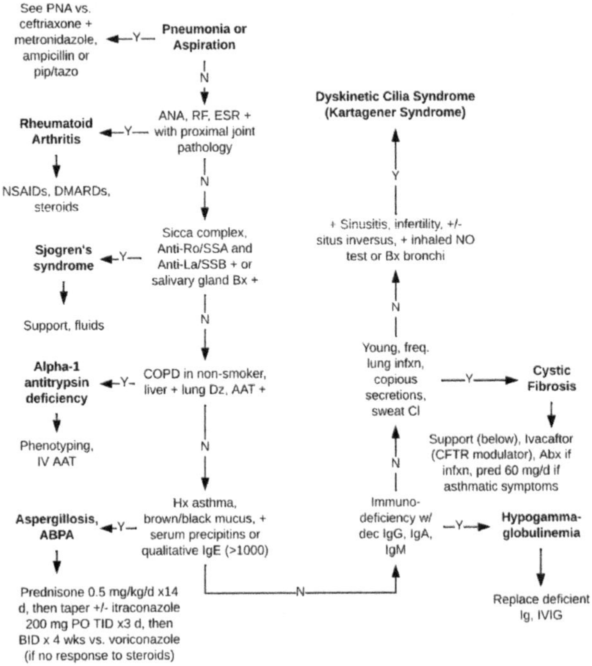

Management

Control Infxn	↓ inflammation	Improve Bronchial Hygiene
- Targeted antibiotic therapy	- Antibiotic therapy - Steroids if ABPA/Asthma - Arformoterol if wheezing	- Turn, cough, deep breathe (TCDB), chest physiotherapy (CPT) - Nebulized hypertonic saline 3 7% BID, albuterol prior to dose to prevent bronchospasm - Inhaled acetylcysteine 3-5 mL 20% or 6-10 mL 10% TID-QID, albuterol prior - Hydration

COPD

<table>
<tr><td rowspan="2">High Risk Airflow Limitation
GOLD 3&4: FEV1 ≤ 50%</td><td colspan="2">Category C</td><td>Category D</td><td rowspan="2">High Risk Exacerbation Hx
≥ 2 AECOPD/1 admit in 12 mo</td></tr>
<tr><td>G1: FEV1 < 50% & <2 AECOPD/yr & no admissions

1st Line: LAMA/LABA

Anoro Ellipta, 1 puff daily

Stiolto Respimat, 2 puffs daily</td><td>G2: Any FEV1 & ≥ 2 AECOPD/yr & ≥ 1 hospitalization

1st Line: ICS/LABA

Symbicort, 2 puff BID

Advair Diskus, 1 puff BID

Breo Ellipta, 1 puff qd</td><td>Many Sx & High Risk for AECOPD

1st Line: ICS/LABA + LAMA

Trelegy Ellipta, 1 puff qd OR

Choice from Cat C, G2 AND

Incruse Ellipta, 1 puff qd

Spiriva (HandiHaler or Respimat), 2 puff daily

Tudorza, 1 puff BID

Consider Daliresp 500 mg PO qd</td></tr>
<tr><td rowspan="2">Low Risk Airflow Limitation
GOLD 1&2: FEV1 ≥ 50%</td><td colspan="2">Category A</td><td>Category B</td><td rowspan="2">Low Risk Exacerbation Hx
1 AECOPD/1 admit in 12 mo</td></tr>
<tr><td colspan="2">Few Sx & Low-risk for AECOPD

1st Line: SABA/SAMA

Albuterol HFA (Proventil, Ventolin, ProAir) 90 mcg 1-2 puffs q4-6h PRN

Levalbuterol HFA (Xopenex) 45 mcg 1-2 puffs q4-6h PRN

Ipratropium HFA (Atrovent) 17 mcg, 2 puff QID, max 12/d

Combivent Respimat, 1 puff QID, max 6/d

DuoNeb, one 3 mL neb q4-6h PRN</td><td>More significant Sx & Low-risk for AECOPD

1st Line: LABA, LAMA/LABA combo

Salmeterol (Serevent Diskus), 1 puff q12h

Arformoterol (Brovana), 1 neb q12h

Formoterol (Perforomist), 1 neb q12h

See Category D for LAMAs

Anoro Ellipta (LAMA/LABA), 1 puff qd

Stiolto Respimat (LAMA/LABA), 2 puffs qd</td></tr>
<tr><td></td><td colspan="2">Less Sx (CAT < 10 & mMRC 0-1)</td><td>Less Sx (CAT ≥ 10 & mMRC ≥2)</td><td></td></tr>
</table>

AECOPD

- Scheduled Albuterol/Ipratropium neb vs. Albuterol q4h + continue home inhalers/nebs
- Steroids
  - Prednisone 40 mg PO daily x 5 d +/- continuation with taper
  - Methylprednisolone 40 mg IV q6h, ?Taper @ D/C
- ↓/avoid BBs
- Antibiotics if change in baseline cough or more productive
  - Azithromycin 500 mg IV/PO daily x5 days
  - Ceftriaxone 1-2g IV daily x 5-7 d
- Supplemental O2, NC vs. NIV if hypercapnic

Asthma

Components of Severity		Classification of Asthma Severity (Youths ≥ 12 years of age & Adults)			
		Intermittent	**Persistent**		
		Impairment	**Mild**	**Mod**	**Severe**
Impairment NL FEV1/FVC: 8-19 y/o 85% 20-39 y/o 80% 40-59 y/o 75% 60-80 y/o 70%	**Symptoms**	≤ 2 days/wk	> 2 days/wk, but not daily	Daily	Throughout the day
	Nighttime Awakenings	≤ 2x/month	3-4x/month	> 1x/wk, but not nightly	Often 7x/wk
	SABA Use for Sx Control	≤ 2 days/wk	2 days/wk, but not daily, & not > 1x/d on any d	Daily	Several times per day
	Interference w/ ADLs	None	Minor limitation	Some limitation	Extremely limited
	Lung Fx	NL FEV1 between exacerbations (FEV1 > 80% predicted, FEV1/FVC NL)	FEV1 ≥ 80% predicted FEV1/FVC NL	FEV1 > 60%, but < 80% predicted FEV1/FVC reduced 5%	FEV1 < 60% predicted FEV1/FVC reduced > 5%
Risk	Exacerbations requiring PO steroids	0-1/year	≥ 2/year		
Treatment Recommendation		SABA PRN (Albuterol)	+ Low-dose ICS (Budesonide, Symbicort, Advair)	Med Dose ICS + LABA	High Dose ICS + LABA +/- omalizumab (IgE level)
				Consider PO steroid taper	
		F/U 2-6 wks, eval level of control & adjust accordingly			

Asthma Exacerbation/Status Asthmaticus

- Explore trigger ?influenza/PNA, etc.
- Scheduled Albuterol/ipratropium q4h + PRN
- Methylprednisolone 125 mg IV x1, then 40 mg IV q6h
- Magnesium 2 g IV x1 dose
- Supplemental O2 → HFNC/Vapotherm (NO CPAP/BiPAP while acute d/t barotrauma/PTX)
- Intubate if change Bx, hypoxemia
- Add Budesonide 0.5-1 mg INH BID
- ↓/avoid BBs

Respiratory Inhalers

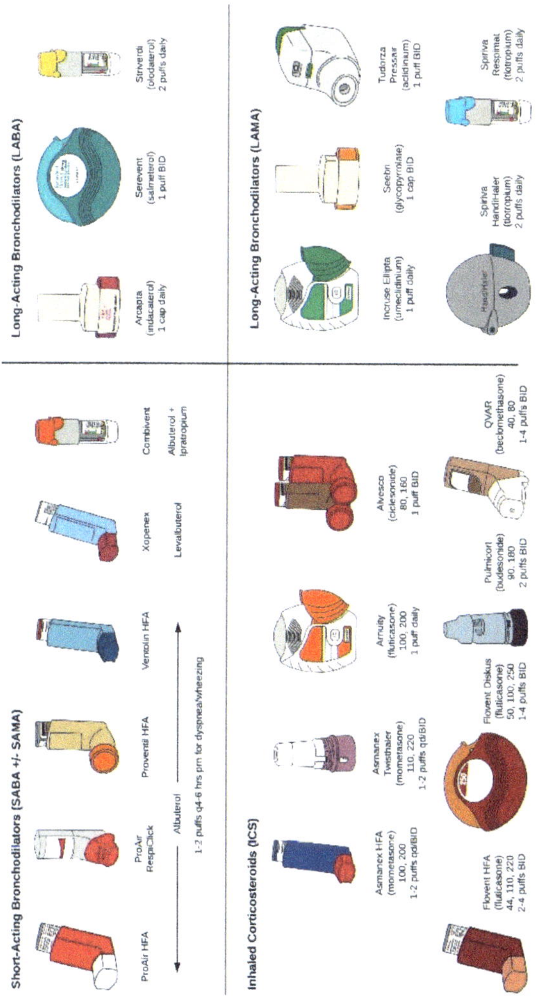

Combination LABA & LAMA

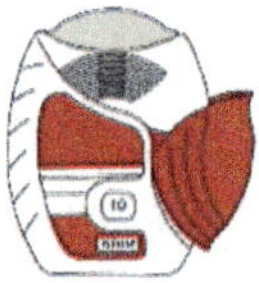

Anoro Ellipta
(umeclidinium &
vilanterol)
1 puff daily

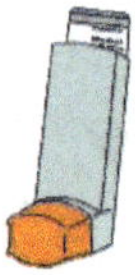

Bevespi
(glycopyrrolate &
formoterol)
2 puffs BID

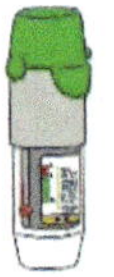

Stiolto Respimat
(olodaterol &
tiotropium)
2 puffs daily

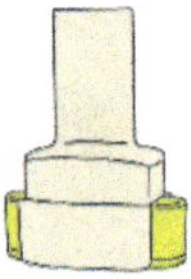

Utibron Neohaler
(indacaterol &
glycopyrrolate)
1 cap BID

Combination LABA & ICS

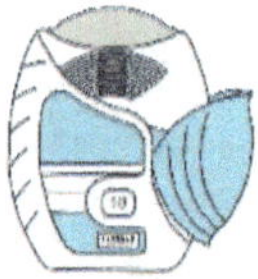

Breo Ellipta
(fluticasone & vilanterol)
100/25, 200/25
1 puff daily

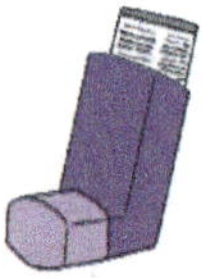

Advair HFA
(fluticasone & salmeterol)
45, 115, 230
2 puffs BID

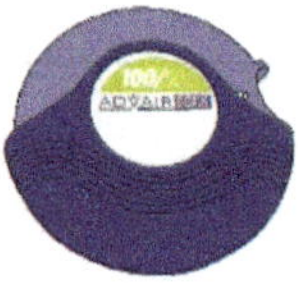

Advair Diskus
(fluticasone & salmeterol)
100, 250, 500
1 puff BID

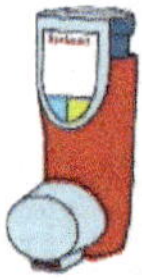

Symbicort
(budesonide & formoterol)
80, 160
2 puffs BID

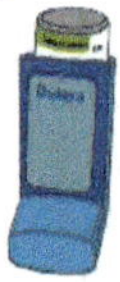

Dulera
(mometasone & formoterol)
100, 200
2 puffs BID

Combination LABA, LAMA, & ICS

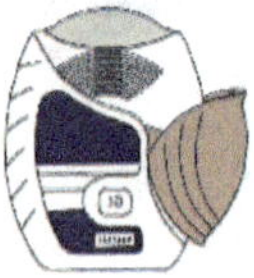

Trelegy Ellipta
(fluticasone,
umeclidinium, &
vilanterol)
100/62.5/25
1 puff daily

Pneumonia (PNA)

Atypical Pneumonia: Systemic symptoms predominate (e.g., fever, malaise, headache). Interstitial/patchy rather than lobular. Often but not always mild. Atypical bacteria (Mycoplasma pneumoniae, Chlamydia pneumoniae, Legionella pneumophilia) (not always)

Evaluation Considerations:

- Empiric Abx for aspiration not recommended
- PCT may be used to de-escalate, but should not be used to determine holding
- Test for pneumococcal (severe PNA) & legionella (outbreak) urine Ags only if indicated
- F/U CXR usually not necessary
- Blood/sputum culture if: severe PNA, Hx MRSA/Pseudomonal infxn, Abx in last 90 days, empiric Rx for MRSA/Pseudomonas
- If cavitary consider TB, fungi, & Nocardia
- If immunocompromised, consider TB, fungi, Nocardia, and PCP
- Steroids only if refractory shock
- Comorbidities = COPD, HF, DM, CA

Prediction Rules	Severe CAP
Tools: CURB-65 (basic) and Pneumonia Severity Index (PSI) (more comprehensive) **Risk Factors:** - Confusion - Uremia (BUN $\geq$ 20 mg/dL) - Respiratory rate $\geq$ 30 - Blood pressure (SBP < 90 or DBP < 60) - Age $\geq$ 65 y/o Few risk factors = outpatient care More risk factors = inpatient versus intensive care unit	1 major and 3 minor criteria Major: - Septic shock - Respiratory failure requiring MV Minor: - RR $\geq$ 30 bpm - $PaO_2/FiO_2 \leq 250$ - Multilobar infiltrates - Confusion - Uremia (BUN $\geq$ 20 mg/dL) - Leukopenia (WBC < 4000 cells/uL) - Thrombocytopenia (plts < 100k cells/uL) - Hypothermia (temp < $36^{\circ}C$) - Hypotension responsive to IVF

	Preferred Option	Additional Considerations
Outpatient No comorbidities	Doxycycline ?Amoxicillin (Doesn't cover atypical)	A macrolide (e.g., Azithromycin) can be used if pneumococcal resistance < 25% (rare)
Outpatient Comorbidities	Amoxicillin/clavulanate OR cephalosporin + macrolide OR doxycycline	Alternative fluoroquinolone (e.g., levofloxacin, moxifloxacin)
Inpatient Non-Severe	Beta-lactam (e.g., ampicillin/sulbactam, ceftriaxone) + macrolide OR fluoroquinolone monotherapy	Add MRSA coverage (e.g., vancomycin or linezolid) +/- pseudomonal coverage (e.g., pip/tazo, cefepime, ceftazidime, imipenem, meropenem, aztreonam) if significant risk factors
Inpatient Severe	Beta-lactam + macrolide OR beta-lactam + fluoroquinolone	

Duration should be 5 days or until clinical resolution (whichever is longer) UNLESS MRSA/pseudomonal pneumonia (7-14 days).

Treatment failure: insufficient time, inadequate antibiotic dose, resistant organism (e.g., MRSA), unusual organism (e.g., GNR, TB, PCP), inadequate source control (e.g., empyema, lung abscess, incorrect diagnosis (e.g., pneumonitis, heart failure, PE, AECOPD).

Tuberculosis

Systemic disease caused by M. Tuberculosis. Pulmonary disease is the most common presentation. Other sites of involvement include lymphatics, genitourinary, bone, meninges, peritoneum, and heart.

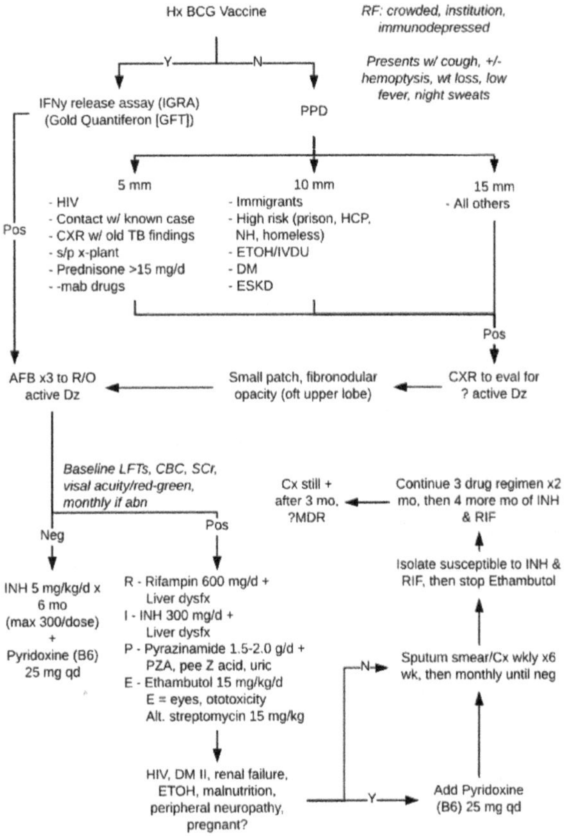

Alveolar Hemorrhage

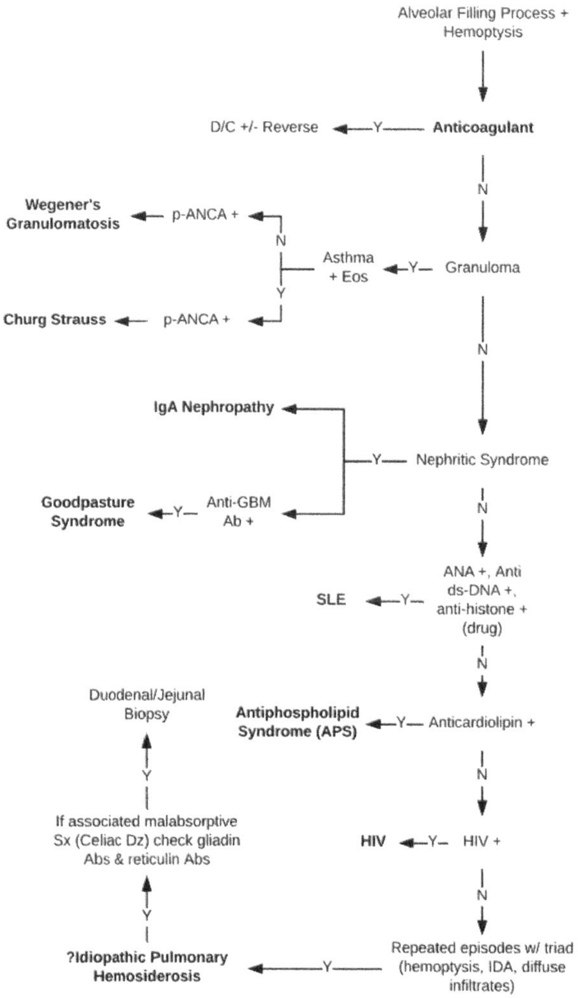

Interstitial Lung Disease (ILD)

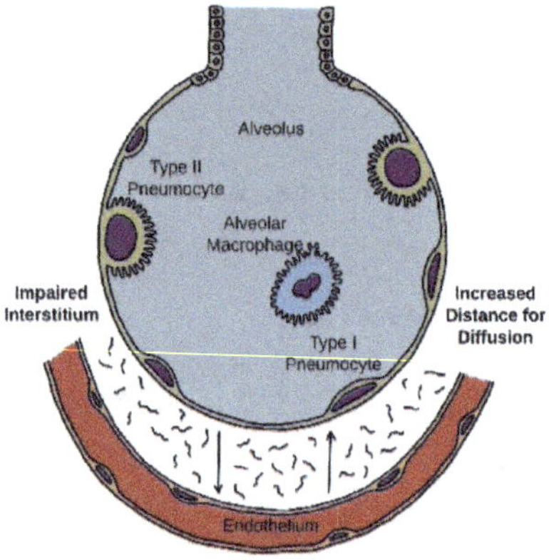

Non-infectious, non-malignant infiltrates of the lung parenchyma (alveoli and interstitium)

Presentation:

- Occupational, environmental, or drug exposure
- Insidious, progressive DOE +/- non-productive +/- clubbing
- Late inspiratory crackles OE
- ↑FEV1/FVC, ↓TLC, FRC, RV
- Reticulonodular pattern on CXR, CT (esp. HRCT) essential for diagnosis

When to Suspect:

- Any patient with "unexplained" dyspnea
- Chronic cough
- Incidental abnormal chest imaging
- Unexplained hypoxia/hypoxemia
- Non-fitting history of "CHF, COPD, recurrent PNA, asthma"

Consider DDx for CXR vs. CT findings

Reticular Pattern	**Cystic Disease**
- Edema: heart failure, pulmonary HTN, TACO, AKI/CKD, hypoalbuminemia - Interstitial pneumonia: viral, PCP, mycoplasma - Lymphangitis carcinomatosis - Interstitial lung disease - Drugs: nitrofurantoin, methotrexate, amiodarone, bleomycin, Cytoxan	- Pulmonary Langerhans cell histiocytosis (PLCH) - Lymphangioleiomyomatosis (LAM) - Pneumatoceles - Lymphocytic interstitial pneumonia **Fine Nodular** - Sarcoidosis - Metastasis - TB

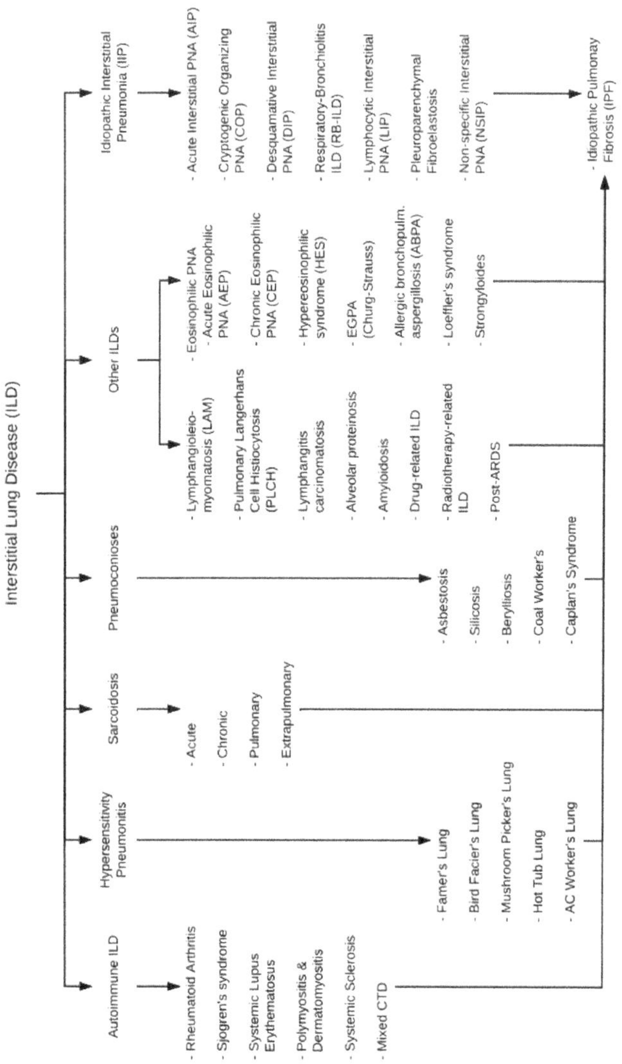

Interstitial Lung Disease (ILD)
Autoimmune ILD
Hypersensitivity Pneumonitis
Sarcoidosis
Pneumoconioses
Other ILDs
Idiopathic Interstitial Pneumonia (IIP)
- Rheumatoid Arthritis
- Sjogren's syndrome
- Systemic Lupus Erythematosus
- Polymyositis & Dermatomyositis
- Systemic Sclerosis
- Mixed CTD
- Famer's Lung
- Bird Facier's Lung
- Mushroom Picker's Lung
- Hot Tub Lung
- AC Worker's Lung
- Acute
- Chronic
- Pulmonary
- Extrapulmonary
- Asbestosis
- Silicosis
- Berylliosis
- Coal Worker's
- Caplan's Syndrome
- Lymphangioleio-myomatosis (LAM)
- Pulmonary Langerhans Cell Histiocytosis (PLCH)
- Lymphangitis carcinomatosis
- Alveolar proteinosis
- Amyloidosis
- Drug-related ILD
- Radiotherapy-related ILD
- Post-ARDS
- Eosinophilic PNA
- Acute Eosinophilic PNA (AEP)
- Chronic Eosinophilic PNA (CEP)
- Hypereosinophilic syndrome (HES)
- EGPA (Churg-Strauss)
- Allergic bronchopulm. aspergillosis (ABPA)
- Loeffler's syndrome
- Strongyloides
- Acute Interstitial PNA (AIP)
- Cryptogenic Organizing PNA (COP)
- Desquamative Interstitial PNA (DIP)
- Respiratory-Bronchiolitis ILD (RB-ILD)
- Lymphocytic Interstitial PNA (LIP)
- Pleuroparenchymal Fibroelastosis
- Non-specific Interstitial PNA (NSIP)
- Idiopathic Pulmonay Fibrosis (IPF)

Autoimmune ILD

Suspect if HRCT with Non-specific interstitial PNA (NSIP) + organizing pneumonia (OP) pattern

Presentation: Insidious & progressive DOE +/- non-productive cough and the following:

Condition	Presentation	Labs
Rheumatoid arthritis	Symmetric arthralgia, am joint stiffness, rheumatoid nodules	ANA, RF, Anti-CCP
Sjogren's Syndrome	Sicca complex (dry eyes, dry mouth), parotid enlargement	ANA, Anti-SSA/Ro, Anti-SSB/La
Systemic Lupus Erythematosus	SOAP: serositis, oral ulcers, arthritis, photosensitivity (4+ Se 85%, Sp 95%)	ANA, Anti-dsDNA (Sp!), ↓ C3 > C4
Polymyositis	Mechanic's hands, proximal muscle weakness	ANA, CK > 10 x NL, Anti-Jo-1
Dermatomyositis	Polymyositis + skin changes, Gottron's papules (Sp!)	ANA, CK, Anti-Jo-1, Anti-Mi-2
Systemic Sclerosis	Raynaud, digital ulcers, GERD, esophageal dysmotility	ANA, RF, Anti-centromere Abs (limited), Anti-RNA polymerase III Abs (diffuse), Anti-SCl-70 (poor prognosis)
Mixed CTD	Mixed features of above	ANA, anti-ribonucleoprotein (RNP) Abs

Hypersensitivity Pneumonitis

Presentation: Exposure (farmer, grain, pet birds, meds, AC, hot tub)

Labs/Imaging: Serum precipitins +, HRCT with homogeneous ground glass opacities

BAL: Lymphocytosis > 50%, CD8 > CD4

Histopathology: Poorly formed granulomas

Rx: Remove offending, steroid +/- azathioprine vs. mycophenolate mofetil to spare steroids

Sarcoidosis

Presentation: > 50 y/o F > M with non-productive cough OR cough w/ clear sputum, tender erythematous nodules, 30-50% extra-pulmonary organ involvement

Labs: Poss. ↑ Ca++ (renal involvement 1-2%), +/- ↑ ACE

CXR/HRCT: Bilat hilar LAD +/- parenchymal or diffuse infiltrates

Histopathology: Non-caseating & non-necrotic granulomas

BAL: CD4 > CD8, lymphocytes ~20%

Rx: Stepwise: steroids —> antimetabolite (e.g., MTX) —> Anti-TNF (e.g., infliximab) —> Additional (Rituximab) —> transplant

Cystic ILDs

Condition	Imaging	Support for Dx
Lymphangio-leiomyomatosis (LAM)	Round, smooth, thin-walled cysts in a diffuse distribution with normal lung parenchyma	Screen for TSC, scan for AMLs, VEGF-D >800 pg/mL (100% Sp), Transbronchial Bx or VATS
Birt-Hogg Dube (DHB)	Lentiform cysts abutting pleura/vessels in a basilar distribution	Family Hx, skin biopsy, FLCN testing, screen for renal tumors
Pulmonary Langerhans Cell Histiocytosis (PLCH)	Bizarre, irregular shaped cysts along with nodules and cavities in an upper lobe distribution	Smoking Hx, DI, bone lesions, transbronchial Bx or VATS, genotyping for MAPK mutations
Lymphocytic interstitial pneumonia (LIP), Follicular Bronchiolitis (FB), Sjogren's	Cysts with wide size variation, eccentric vessels, dissolving lung, ground glass opacities, nodules	Sicca symptoms, SS-A, SS-B, ANA, RF, VATS Bx
Consider Alpha-1 antitrypsin (AAT) deficiency & emphysema, paraseptal emphysema (almost imperceptible walls), honeycombing (uniform rows), cyst (thin < 2 mm wall). If no wall, then likely centrilobular emphysema. Thicker wall likely abscess.		

Eosinophilic

Allergic Bronchopulmonary Aspergillosis (ABPA)	Loeffler's Syndrome
Presentation: Hx CF > asthma w/ dyspnea, fever, cough productive of black/brown mucus. **Labs**: AEC > 500 cells/uL, + Aspergillus skin test OR IgE against A. Fumigatus, IgE > 1000, Serum precipitins to aspergillus **Imaging**: Finger-in-glove w/ bronchiectasis, upper lobe predominance +/- tree-in-bud **Rx**: Steroids, add itraconazole or vorconazole if unable to taper steroids	**Presentation**: Immigrant from Cuba or Dominican Republic w/ non-productive cough, dyspnea, substernal burning provoked by cough. **Labs**: AEC > 1,500 cells/uL (>10%) **Imaging**: Transient or fleeting pulmonary opacities, round/oval, migratory **BAL**: Eos > 25%
Strongyloidiasis	**Acute Eosinophilic Pneumonia (AEP)**
Presentation: Hx HIV, drugs, x-plant, malnutrition +/- asthma recently immigrated from Latin America w/ years of pulmonary (cough, dyspnea, +/- hemoptysis), GI (duodenitis), and skin (pruritic skin lesions). **Labs**: Eosinophils in both lung & blood **Imaging**: Round infiltrates c/w foci of hemorrhage, pneumonitis, and edema **Rx**: Ivermectin > Albendazole	**Presentation**: 20-40 y/o M > F (2x) smoker who recently quit +/- Hx allergic Dz presents w/ non-productive cough, SOB, fever < 4 wks **Labs**: Neutrophilic leukocytosis; Eos in lung, not blood; $\uparrow$ CRP/ESR; $\uparrow$ IgE & IL-5 **Imaging**: BL, random, patchy, ground glass or reticular opacities +/- centrilobular nodules **BAL**: > 25% Eos **Rx**: Supportive care, empiric Abx until cultures, steroids, smoking cessation

Chronic Eosinophilic Pneumonia (CEP)	Eosinophilic Granulomatosis with Polyangiitis (EGPA)
Presentation: 30-40 y/o M > F (2x) with Hx asthma 50% OR atopy 60% presents with gradual onset non-productive cough, low fever, night sweats, wt loss over 1-4 mo **Labs**: Eos in both lung & blood (> 6%, >1000/uL), ↑ IgE (50% pts), IL-5, high ESR/CRP **Imaging**: Photographic negative of pulmonary edema (very peripheral BL/pleural-based infiltrates) **BAL**: Eos ≥ 25% **Rx**: Steroids (Prednisone 0.5 mg/kg/d OR methylprednisolone 250 mg IV q6h x 3 d), inhaled beclomethasone, smoking cessation	**Presentation**: Male > female with Hx asthma 10 yrs + sinusitis (+/- addition of LTRA [montelukast] correlating with symptom onset) presents with dyspnea + Vasculitic – purpura, mononeuritis multiplex **Labs**: AEC > 1,500 cells/uL, ANCA + 50% pts, +/- ↑ IgE **Imaging**: Transient and patchy opacities with lobar or segmental distribution **BAL**: Eos > 25% **Rx**: Steroids, CYP, MTX, therapeutic plasmapheresis, mepolizumab

Idiopathic Interstitial Pneumonias (IIPs)

Condition	Histo Pattern	Radiology	Distribution	CT Findings
IPF	UIP	Basal-predominant reticular abnormality w/ volume loss	Peripheral, subpleural, basal	Reticular, honeycombing, traction bronchiectasis, architectural distortion, focal GGO
NSIP	NSIP	GGO and reticular opacities	Subpleural, peribronchial	GGO, irregular lines, consolidation
COP	OP	Patchy bilat consolidation	Subpleural/ peribronchial	Patchy consolidation +/- nodules
AIP	DAD	Progressive diffuse GGO	Diffuse	Consolidation & GGO, often lobular sparing, traction bronchiectasis later
DIP	DIP	GGO	Lower zone, peripheral predominance mostly	GGO, reticular lines
RB-ILD	RB	Bronchial wall thickening; GGO	Diffuse	Bronchial wall thickening, centrilobular nodules, patchy GGO
LIP	LIP	Reticular opacities, nodules	Diffuse	Centrilobular nodules, GGO, septal and bronchovascular thickening, thin-walled cysts

Pleural Fluid Analysis

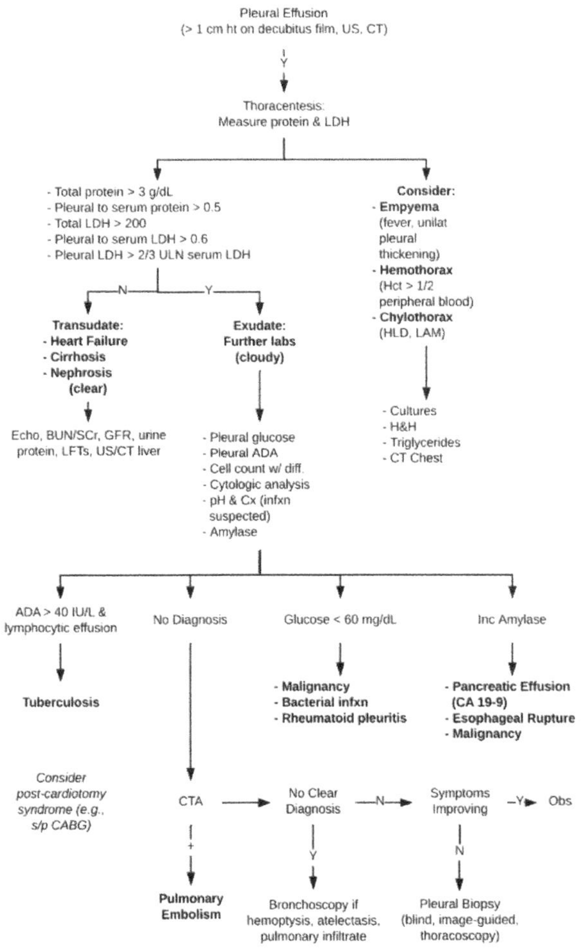

Effusion Rx: Metolazone 5-20 mg PO (block Na receptors), wait 30 min, give Lasix 40-80 mg IV

Pulmonary Hypertension

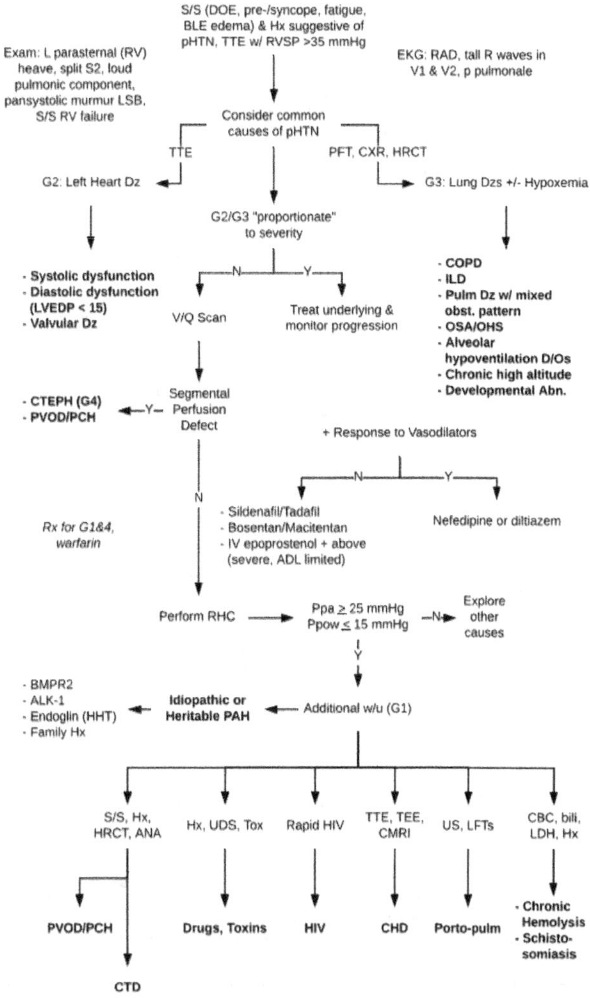

Oxygen Modalities

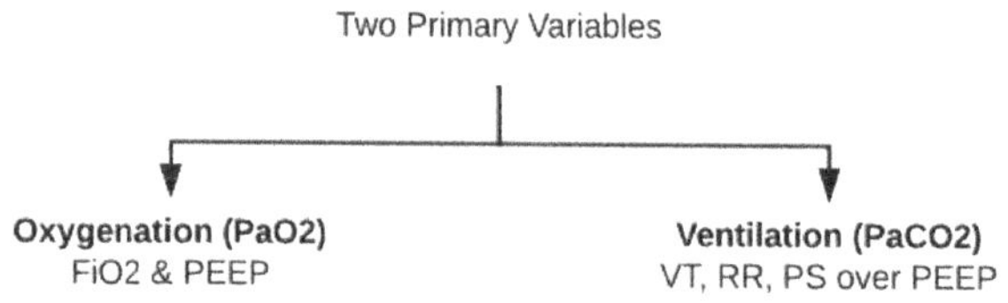

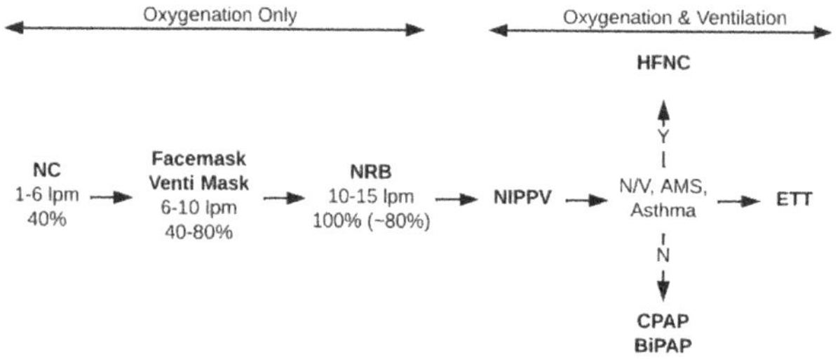

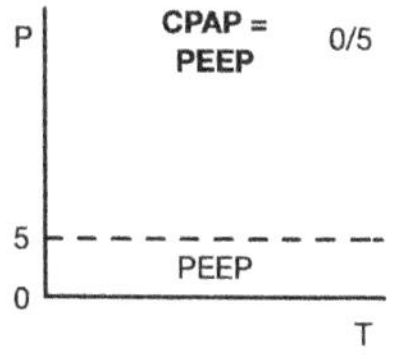

Primarily OSA

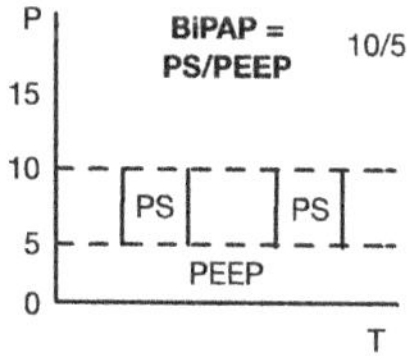

COPD, but not
asthma b/c
barotrauma

Rapid Sequence Induction (RSI)

1 Prepare

Indications:

- Airway protection
- Respiratory failure
- O2 consumption > delivery
- Secondary brain injury prevention, terminate seizure
- Temperature control
- Humanitarian (procedure)

→

LEMON

L - Look @ Anatomy
E - Evaluate 3-3-2
M - Mallampati
O - Obstruction?
N - Neck Mobility

→

I - Informed Consent
S - Suction
O - Oxygen
A - Airway Equipment
P - Pharm Agents
M - Monitor
E - ETCO2

---

2 Pre-Oxygenate

100% NRB for 3-5 min + 15 L/NC → Nitrogen washout, prevents prolonged desaturation

---

3 Pre-Medicate

Analgesia → Sedation → Paralysis

Analgesia:
Fentanyl 1-5 mcg/kg

Sedation:

- HD Stable
  - Midazolam 0.05-0.1 mg/kg
  - Propofol 0.5-1 mg/kg
- HD Unstable
  - Etomidate 0.03-0.1 mg/kg
  - Ketamine 1-2 mg/kg

Paralysis:

NOT IF: Hyperthermic, hyperkalemic b/c rhabdo & shock

Succinylcholine 0.6 mg/kg (up to 150 mg)

Rocuronium 0.6-1.2 mg/kg

- Atropine gtts to dry the airway
- Zofran/Phenergan for nausea

---

4 Pass the Tube

Cormack-Lehane Scale

---

5 Proof of Placement

(1) Visualize through the vocal cords
(2) Bilateral breath sounds
(3) No epigastric sounds
(4) ETCO2, YELLOW
(5) CXR 2 cm above carina

---

6 Post-Intubation Management

F - Feeding/Fluids
A - Analgesia
S - Sedation
T - Thromboprophylaxis
H - HOB 30 degrees
U - Ulcer prophylaxis
G - Glycemic control

Intubation & Mechanical Ventilation

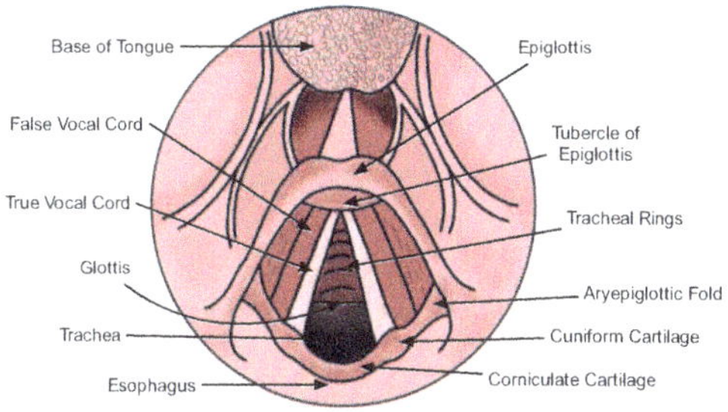

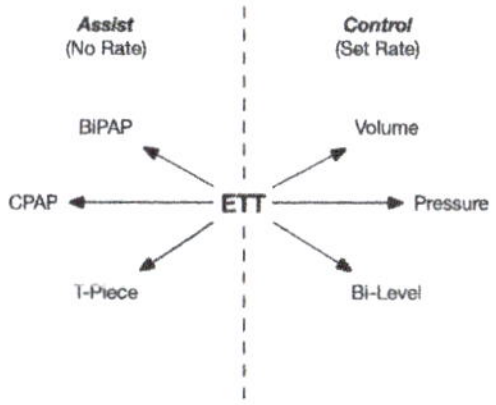

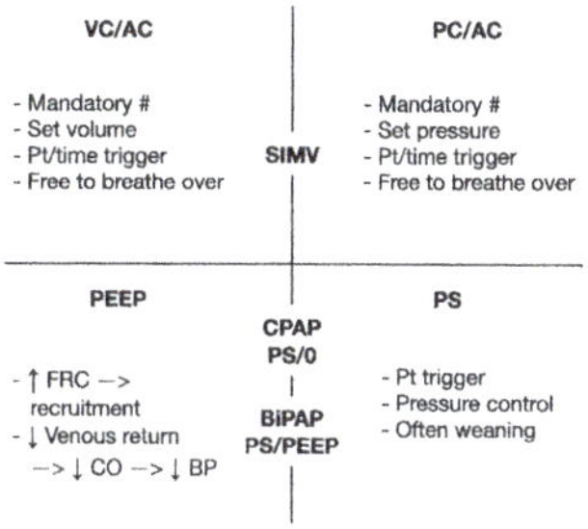

Ventilation (PaCO2)			Oxygenation (PaO2)	
Rate	VT	Flow Rate (IFR)	FiO2	PEEP
12-16 BPM	6-8 mL/kg PBW ~500-600	60+ L/min	Start 100%, titrate	5-24 cm H2O
Barotrauma, autoPEEP & air trapping → ↓ venous return, impede exp. & spontaneous vent	Volutrauma PBW: Male = 50 +2.3 (ht in – 60) Female = 45.5 + 2.3 (ht in – 60)	Comfort; Controls how quickly air goes in	Mitochondrial dysFx d/t ROS & ↓ NO → absorption atelectasis → shunt → hypoxemia	VILI, ↓ venous return → ↓ CO → HoTN

Mechanical Ventilation Strategies

Obstructive (Asthma/COPD)

Give as much expiratory time as possible

- Mode: Assist control
- Vt: 8 mL/kg PBW
- IFR: 80-100 lpm
- PEEP: 0
- FiO2: 30-100%
- RR: Start @ 10, titrate to I:E 1:4 or 1:5
- Allow for permissive hypercapnia w/ pH 7.1
    - May need sedation/opioids/bicarb gtt
- Avoid AutoPEEP & air trapping w/ above

Injury (all other pts)

- Mode: Assist control
- Vt (protection): 6-8 mL/kg PBW, goal 6 mL/kg (leave alone)
- IFR (comfort): 60-80 lpm, ↑ if "sucking through straw"
- RR: start 18, adjust per CO2, allow permissive hypercapnia
- FiO2 & PEEP: Start 100% w/ PEEP 5, check ABG 5 min, set FiO2 to 30%, then titrate per chart below (q5-10 min, quicker if low SpO2)
- Goal: PaO2 55-80 mmHg or SpO2 88-95%
- Plateau pressure: check after initial settings then regular intervals using inspiratory hold button, hold for 0.5 sec, look @ pressure
    - Maintain < 30 cm H2O, lower Vt by 1 mL/kg
        - May need as low as 4 mL/kg
    - If Pplat < 25 & Vt < 6, ↑ Vt by 1 mL/kg

Lower PEEP/Higher FiO2:

FiO2	0.3	0.4	0.4	0.5	0.5	0.6	0.7
PEEP	5	5	8	8	10	10	10

FiO2	0.7	0.7	0.8	0.9	0.9	0.9	1.0
PEEP	12	14	14	14	16	18	18-24

Higher PEEP/Lower FiO2:

FiO2	0.3	0.3	0.3	0.3	0.3	0.4	0.4
PEEP	5	8	10	12	14	14	16

FiO2	0.5	0.5	0.5-0.8	0.8	0.9	1.0	1.0
PEEP	16	18	20	22	22	22	24

Ventilator Alarm Analysis

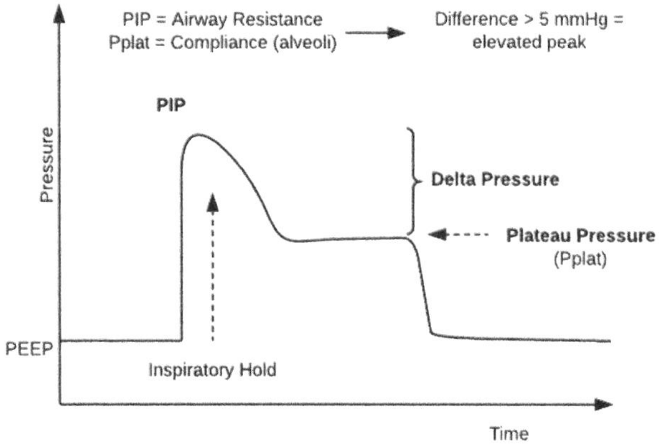

D: Displacement, right mainstem/dislodgement
O: Obstruction, mucous plug, tubing kink, tight airways
P: Pneumothorax, get CXR
E: Equipment failure, disconnect and use BVM w/ PEEP valve
R: Rigidity of chest wall s/t fentanyl (Rx BZDs, naloxone, NMB)

High Pressure Alarm (10-15 cm H2O > PIP)

Peak = Resistance

- Bronchospasm or bronchoconstriction (nebs, steroids)
- Secretions or mucus plug (suction)
- ETT/circuitry kinked/biting (fix, bite block)
- Asynchronous breathing (↑sedation/analgesia)

Plateau = Compliance

- Get a CXR
- PTX
- Pulmonary edema
- ARDS
- Pneumonia
- ADHF
- Pulmonary hemorrhage
- Pleural effusion

Low Pressure Alarm (5-10 cm H2O < PIP)

Inability to build up airway pressure b/c disconnection, leak, cuff deflation OR change in compliance/resistance

Low VT/VE

Not getting out what you put in d/t cuff deflation/herniation above cord, bronchopleural fistula

Low O_2 alarm: O_2 not attached to wall/plugged in wrong

Cardiology

Chest Pain

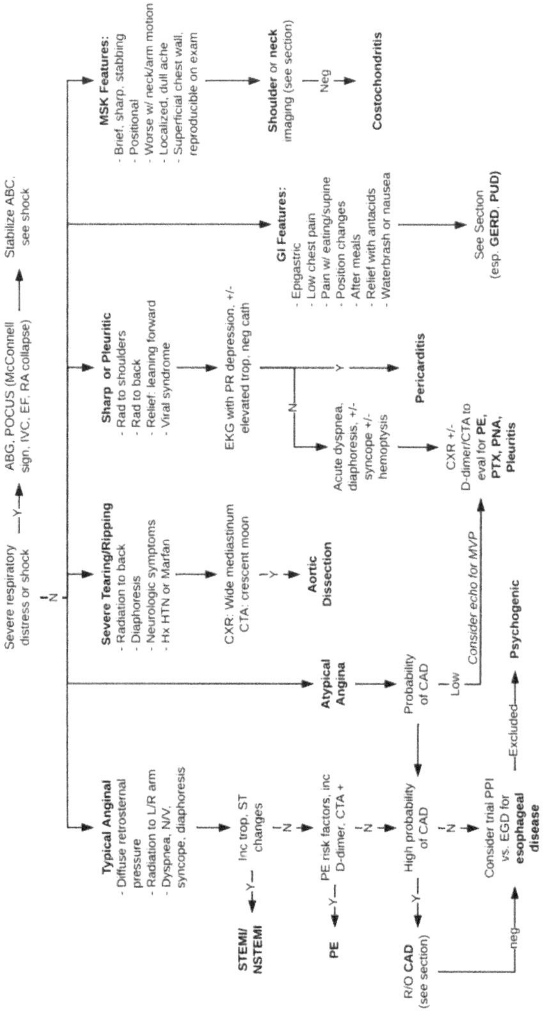

Severe respiratory distress or shock
Y
ABG, POCUS (McConnell sign, IVC, EF, RA collapse)
Stabilize ABC, see shock
N
Typical Anginal
- Diffuse retrosternal pressure
- Radiation to L/R arm
- Dyspnea, N/V, syncope, diaphoresis
Atypical Angina
Severe Tearing/Ripping
- Radiation to back
- Diaphoresis
- Neurologic symptoms
- Hx HTN or Marfan
Sharp or Pleuritic
- Rad to shoulders
- Rad to back
- Relief: leaning forward
- Viral syndrome
GI Features:
- Epigastric
- Low chest pain
- Pain w/ eating/supine
- Position changes
- After meals
- Relief with antacids
- Waterbrash or nausea
MSK Features:
- Brief, sharp, stabbing
- Positional
- Worse w/ neck/arm motion
- Localized, dull ache
- Superficial chest wall, reproducible on exam
Inc trop, ST changes
Y
STEMI/ NSTEMI
N
PE risk factors, inc D-dimer, CTA +
Y
PE
N
High probability of CAD
Y
R/O CAD (see section)
N
Consider trial PPI vs. EGD for esophageal disease
neg
Excluded
Psychogenic
Probability of CAD
Low
Consider echo for MVP
CXR: Wide mediastinum CTA: crescent moon
Y
Aortic Dissection
EKG with PR depression, +/- elevated trop, neg cath
Y
Pericarditis
N
Acute dyspnea, diaphoresis, +/- syncope +/- hemoptysis
CXR +/- D-dimer/CTA to eval for PE, PTX, PNA, Pleuritis
See Section (esp. GERD, PUD)
Shoulder or neck imaging (see section)
Neg
Costochondritis

Palpitations

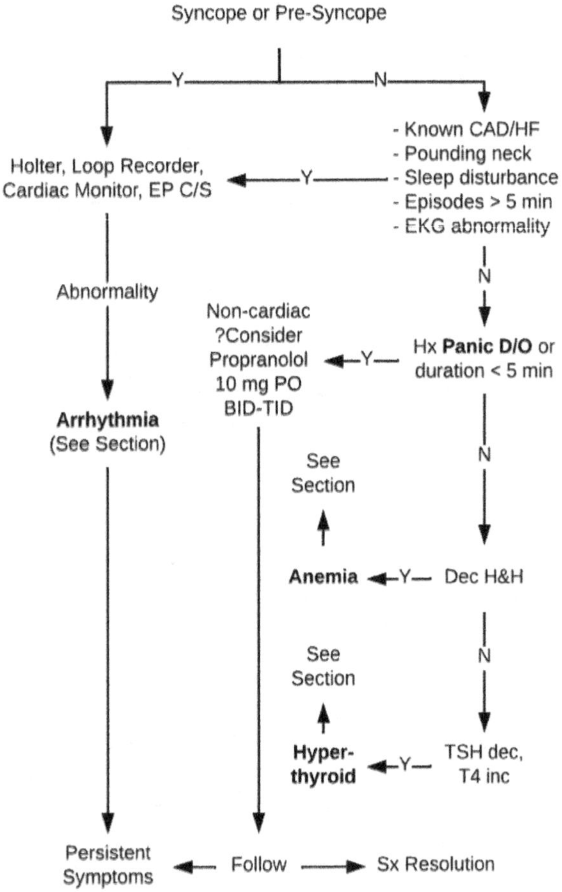

Edema

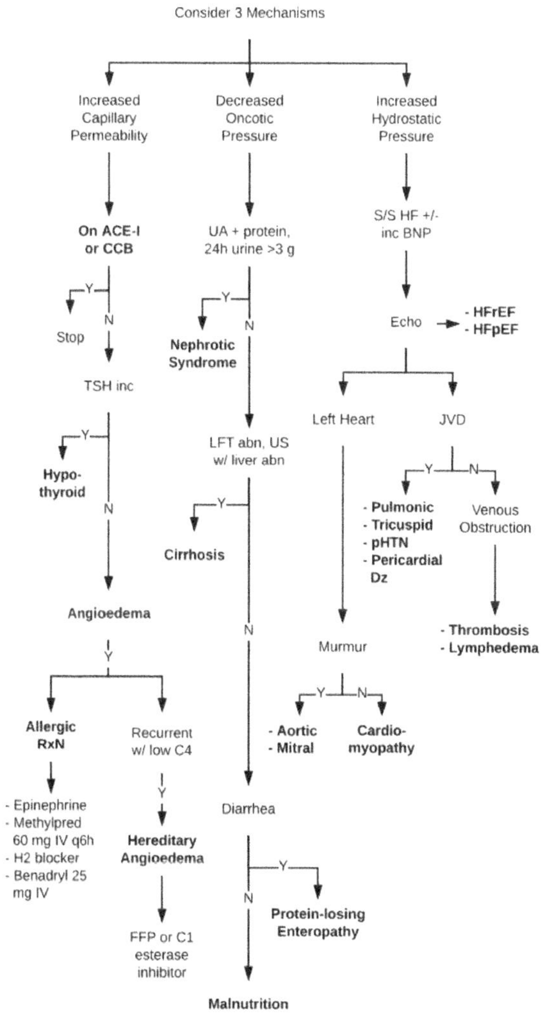

Consider 3 Mechanisms
Increased Capillary Permeability
Decreased Oncotic Pressure
Increased Hydrostatic Pressure
On ACE-I or CCB
Y
Stop
N
TSH inc
Y
Hypo-thyroid
N
Angioedema
Y
Allergic RxN
- Epinephrine
- Methylpred 60 mg IV q6h
- H2 blocker
- Benadryl 25 mg IV
Recurrent w/ low C4
Y
Hereditary Angioedema
FFP or C1 esterase inhibitor
UA + protein, 24h urine >3 g
Y
Nephrotic Syndrome
N
LFT abn, US w/ liver abn
Y
Cirrhosis
N
Diarrhea
Y
Protein-losing Enteropathy
N
Malnutrition
S/S HF +/- inc BNP
Echo
- HFrEF
- HFpEF
Left Heart
Murmur
Y
N
- Aortic
- Mitral
Cardio-myopathy
JVD
Y
N
- Pulmonic
- Tricuspid
- pHTN
- Pericardial Dz
Venous Obstruction
- Thrombosis
- Lymphedema

Echocardiogram

Normal		**Aortic Valve**	
Aortic annulus size	1.8 – 2.3 cm	Normal area	2.5 – 4.5 cm^2
Mitral annulus size	3.0 – 3.5 cm	Mild stenosis	1.0 – 2.5 cm^2
Aortic VTI	18 – 25 cm	Moderate stenosis	0.75 – 1.0 cm^2
Mitral VTI	10 – 13 cm	Severe stenosis	< 0.75 cm^2
Mitral Valve		**Aortic Valve Mean Gradient**	
Normal area	4.0 – 4.6 cm^2	Normal gradient	< 5 mmHg
Mild stenosis	1.5 – 2.5 cm^2	Mild stenosis	5 – 25 mmHg
Moderate stenosis	1.0 – 1.5 cm^2	Moderate stenosis	25 – 50 mmHg
Severe stenosis	< 1.0 cm^2	Severe stenosis	> 50 mmHg
Mitral Valve Mean Gradient		**Aortic Peak Gradient**	
Normal gradient	< 2 mmHg	Normal gradient	< 16 mmHg
Mild stenosis	2 – 6 mmHg	Mild stenosis	16 – 36 mmHg
Moderate stenosis	6 – 12 mmHg	Moderate stenosis	36 – 75 mmHg
Severe stenosis	> 12 mmHg	Severe stenosis	> 75 mmHg
Aortic Regurgitation PHT		**Pulmonary HTN (Peak Pressure)**	
Mild AR	> 550 msec	Mild	30 – 40 mmHg
Moderate AR	300 – 550 msec	Moderate	40 – 70 mmHg
Severe AR	< 300 msec	Severe	> 70, PAP > 40
Aortic Regurgitation DT		**dP/dt**	
Mild AR	< 2.0 m/sec	Normal	> 1200 mmHg/s
Moderate AR	2.0 – 3.5 m/sec	Borderline	1000 – 2000
Severe AR	> 3.5 m/sec	Abnormal	< 1000 mmHg/s
AR Jet Diameter/LVOT Ratio		**Index of Myocardial Performance**	
Mild AR	< 25 – 45%	Normal	< 0.40
Moderate AR	45 – 65%	Mildly depressed	0.40 – 0.60
Severe AR	> 65%	Mod. Depressed	0.60 – 1.00
Aortic Regurgitant Fraction		Severely depressed	> 1.00
Normal/Trivial	< 20%		
Mild	20 – 30%		
Moderate	30 – 55%		
Severe	> 55%		
Aortic Regurgitation Vena Contracta			
Mild AR	< 0.3 cm		
Moderate AR	0.3 – 0.6 cm		
Severe AR	> 0.6 cm		

RVSP > 35 mmHg concerning for pulmonary HTN

RVSP 40 mmHg = mPAP 25 mmHg (mPAP ≥ 25 mmHg meets diagnostic criteria for pHTN)

Hyperlipidemia/Atherosclerosis

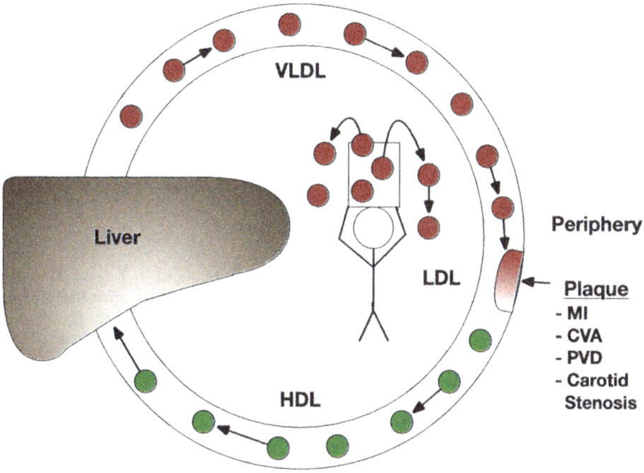

CRP – likelihood of plaque rupture, released by unstable plaque

Lipid Panel

LDL	HDL	TG	Total Cholesterol
< 100 / < 70 if high-risk	< 40 (male) low	< 150 NL	< 200 NL
100 – 129 above	< 50 (female) low	150 – 199 border	200 – 239 border
130 – 159 borderline		200 – 249 high	> 240 high
160 – 189 high		> 500 very high	
> 190 very high			

ASCVD Risk Factors

- Hx ACS (esp. past 12 mo)
- Hx ischemic CVA
- PVD w/ claudication, ABI < 0.85, or previous revascularization/ amputation
- Age > 65 y/o
- Heterozygous familial HLD
- Hx CABG or PCI
- Diabetes mellitus
- Hypertension
- Smoker
- CKD w/ GFR 15-59
- Persistently elevated LDL >100 mg/dL despite max statin and ezetimibe
- Hx heart failure
- TG > 175 mg/mL
- Hx RA, psoriasis, HIV
- CRP > 2.0 mg/L
- Lp(a) > 50 mg/dL
- ApoB > 130 mg/dL
- ABI < 0.9

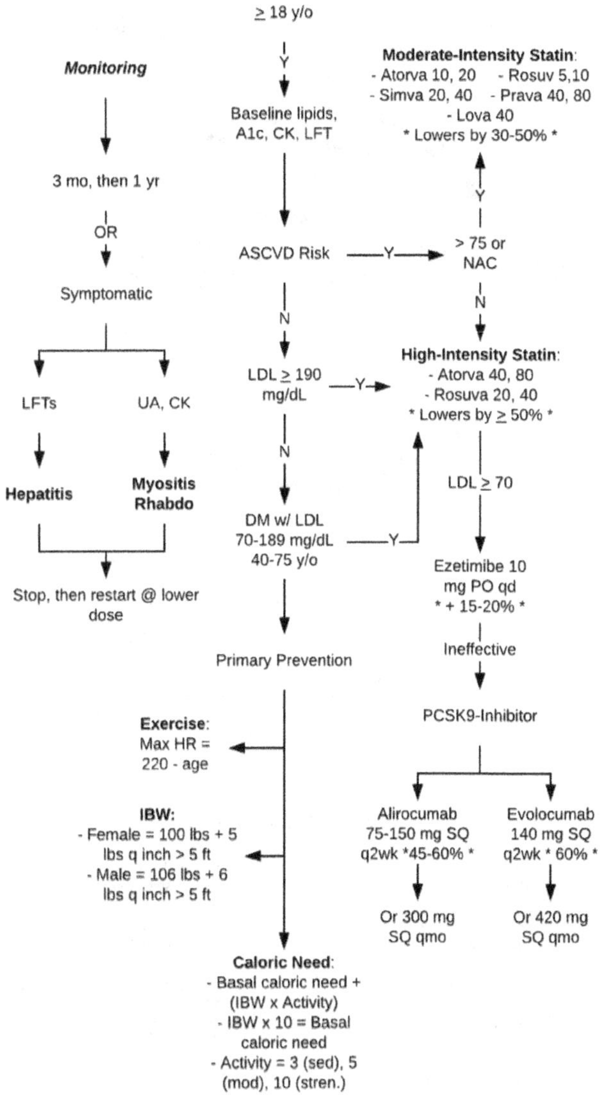

≥ 18 y/o
Y
Baseline lipids, A1c, CK, LFT
ASCVD Risk
Y
> 75 or NAC
Y
Moderate-Intensity Statin:
- Atorva 10, 20 - Rosuv 5,10
- Simva 20, 40 - Prava 40, 80
- Lova 40
* Lowers by 30-50% *
N
N
LDL ≥ 190 mg/dL
Y
High-Intensity Statin:
- Atorva 40, 80
- Rosuva 20, 40
* Lowers by ≥ 50% *
N
DM w/ LDL 70-189 mg/dL 40-75 y/o
Y
LDL ≥ 70
Ezetimibe 10 mg PO qd
* + 15-20% *
Ineffective
PCSK9-Inhibitor
Alirocumab 75-150 mg SQ q2wk *45-60% *
Evolocumab 140 mg SQ q2wk * 60% *
Or 300 mg SQ qmo
Or 420 mg SQ qmo
Primary Prevention
Exercise: Max HR = 220 - age
IBW:
- Female = 100 lbs + 5 lbs q inch > 5 ft
- Male = 106 lbs + 6 lbs q inch > 5 ft
Caloric Need:
- Basal caloric need + (IBW x Activity)
- IBW x 10 = Basal caloric need
- Activity = 3 (sed), 5 (mod), 10 (stren.)
Monitoring
3 mo, then 1 yr
OR
Symptomatic
LFTs
UA, CK
Hepatitis
Myositis Rhabdo
Stop, then restart @ lower dose

Hypertension

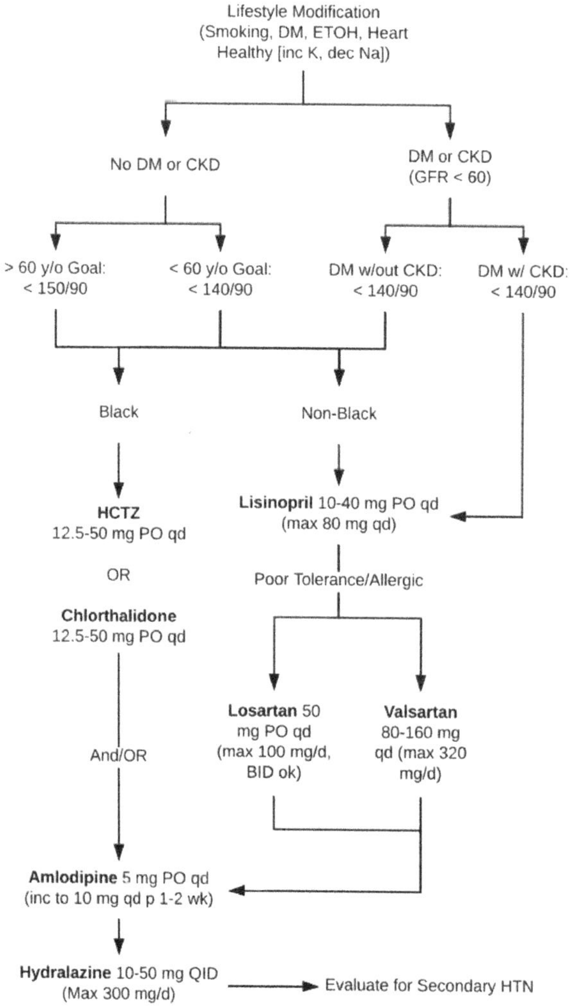

JNC 8

Hypertensive Urgency & Emergency

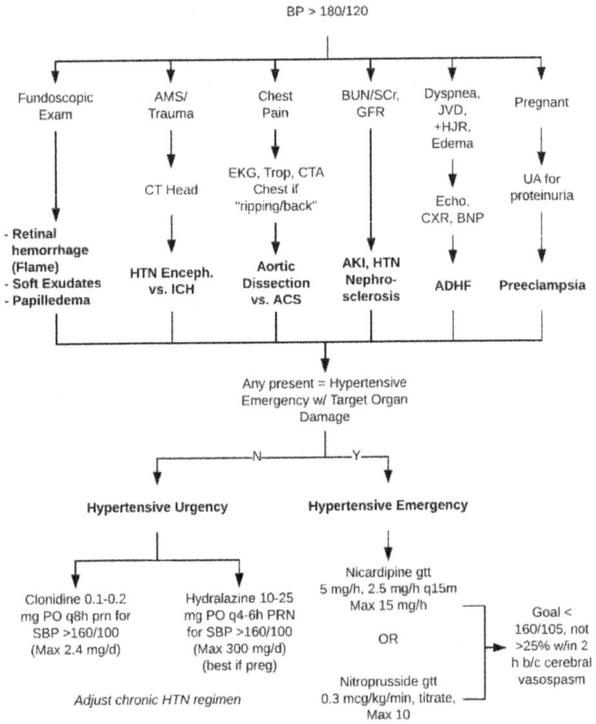

Secondary Hypertension

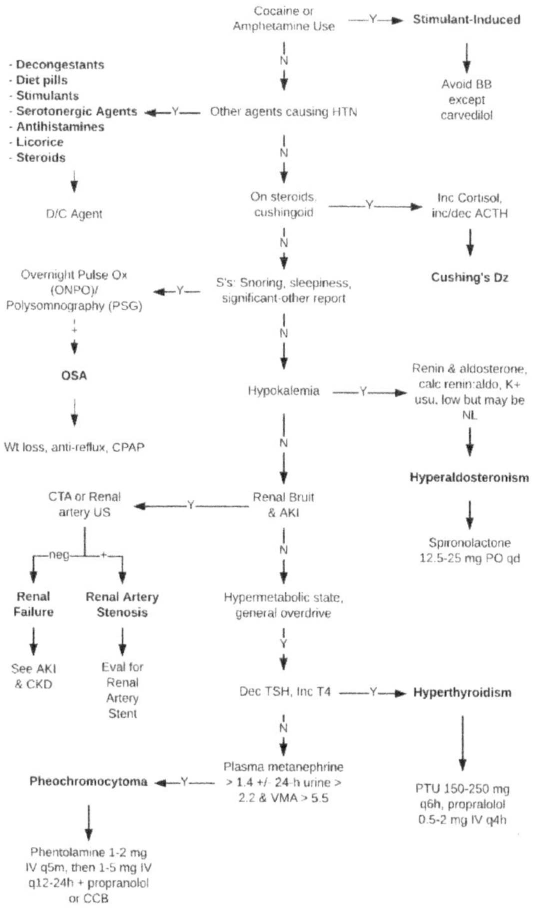

Pericardial Effusion

Accumulation of fluid in pericardial cavity. Ventricular interdependence (change in pressure/volume/function in one ventricle influences the function of the other)

Etiology (based on fluid analysis):
- Exudative – pericarditis, CV Sx, chemo, infxn, AI (SLE)
- Transudative – LHF, FVO, hypoproteinemia
- Serosanguinous – TB, neoplasm, uremia, radiation
- Frank blood – aortic root dissection, free wall rupture, trauma, coagulopathy

Manifestations:
- CP relieved by sitting up & forward, worse supine
- Lightheadedness
- Syncope
- Palpitations
- Cough
- Dyspnea

PEx:
- Ewart sign – dull percussion beneath L scapula
- Tachycardia, tachypnea, fever
- Beck's triad if tamponade
- Pericardial friction rub if pericarditis
- Diminished breath sounds if effusion

Dx: CXR with "water bottle" sign, echo with evidence of effusion

DDx: acute pericarditis, tamponade, cardiogenic pulmonary edema, DCM, MI, PE

Rx:
- Pericardiocentesis for DDx
- Target etiology
- ASA/NSAIDs
- Colchicine
- Steroids
- Abx if indicated

Echo: Effusion

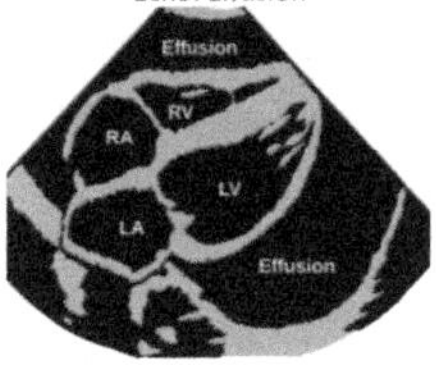

Cardiac Tamponade

Pericardial effusion → cardiac compression; where pericardial pressure > intracardiac pressure (not always hypotensive, but always tachycardic)

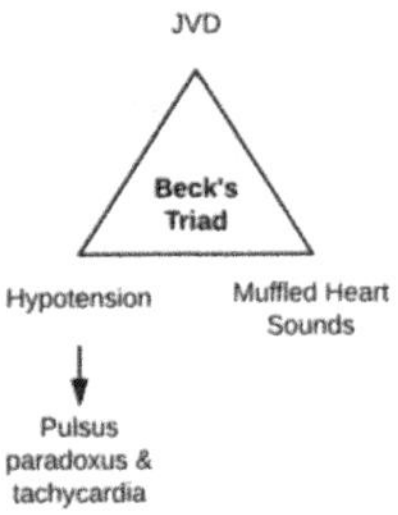

EKG: QRS alternans, low voltage, tachycardia

Echocardiogram:
- ↑ pericardial fluid
- RA and RV collapse
- Abnormal motion of the septum
- IVC distention without normal collapse during inspiration
- Swinging heart b/c the heart is free floating in pericardial fluid

Management: NSAIDs, steroids, target etiology, pericardiocentesis, pericardial window

Coronary Artery Disease (CAD)

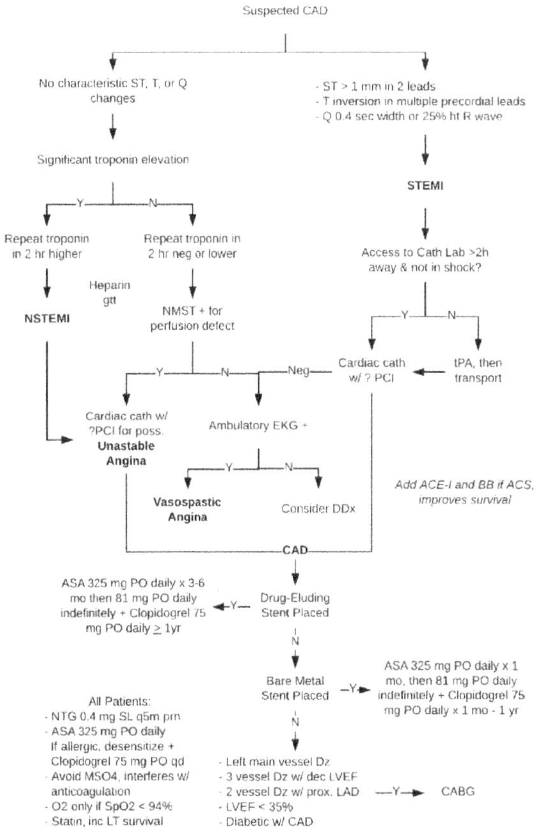

MI Location	Coronary Artery	Leads
Inferior	Right Circumflex Artery (RCA)	II, III, aVF
Septal	Left Anterior Descending (LAD)	V1-V2
Anterior	LAD	V3-V4
Lateral	LAD &/or Left Circumflex	V5-V6, I, aVL
Anterolateral	LAD	V1-V6
Posterior	RCA or Posterior Descending (PD)	V1-V2, larger R than septal
Right Ventricle (Right-Side EKG)	RCA	V1, V3r, V4r

I Lateral	aVR	V1 septal	V4 Anterior
II Inferior	aVL Lateral	V2 Septal	V5 Lateral
III Inferior	aVF Inferior	V3 Anterior	V6 Lateral

Enzyme	Onset	Peak	Duration	Specificity
Myoglobin	Immediate	1-4 h	24 h	Best if day of CP
CK-MB	4-6 h	12-24 h	3-4 d	SM Injury
CK-MB2	2-3 h	6-9 h	3-4 d	SM Injury
Troponin I	4-6 h	24 h	10-14 d	*Most spec*
Troponin T	4-6 h	24 h	10-14 d	CKD etc.

Troponinemia DDx:

- Pericarditis
- Myocarditis
- Cardiac contusion/trauma
- Renal failure
- Extreme exertion
- LVH
- Endocarditis
- Aortic dissection
- Pulmonary embolism
- Shock state/critical illness
- Peripheral arterial Dz
- Coronary vasospasm
- HOCM
- Stroke
- Defibrillation/CPR
- Chronic severe HF
- Cardiac arrhythmia
- Burns

Who is at Risk for ACS?

- Typical CP Findings
- ST-deviation
- Non-specific repolarization disturbance
- Advanced age, esp. > 65 y/o
- Hx HLD, HTN, DM, smoking, obesity
- Family history CAD/SCD
- Trop > 1-3 x ULN

Available Risk Calculators: HEART Score, TIMI, GRACE

ACS Complications

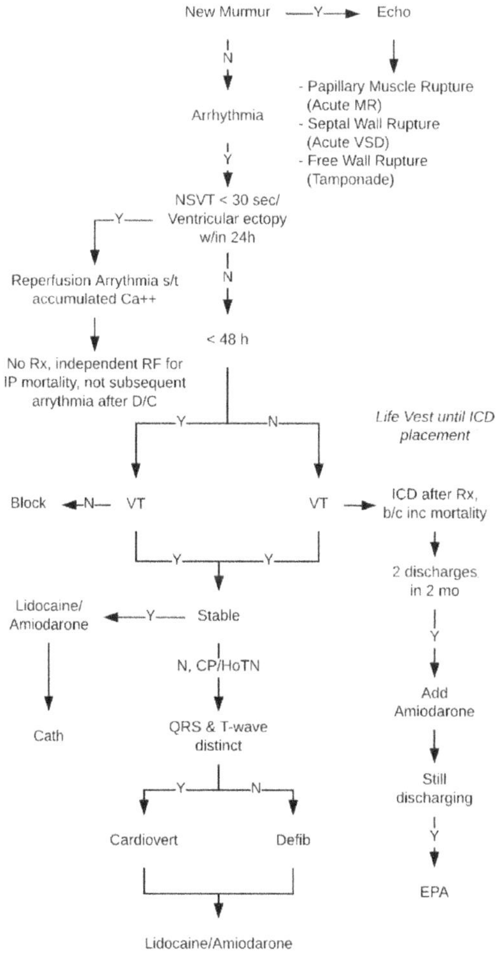

Heart Failure

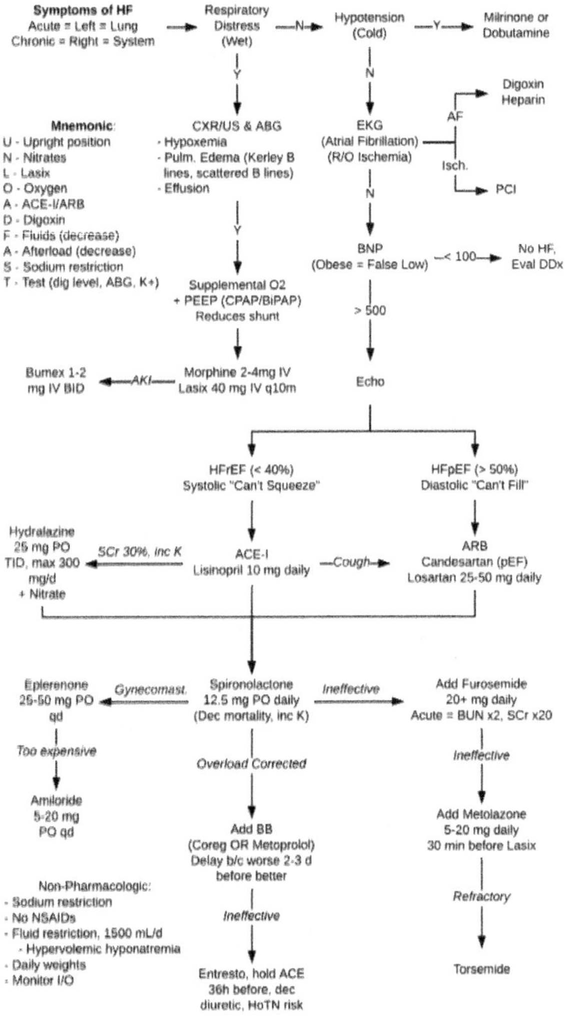

Valvulopathies

Aortic Stenosis

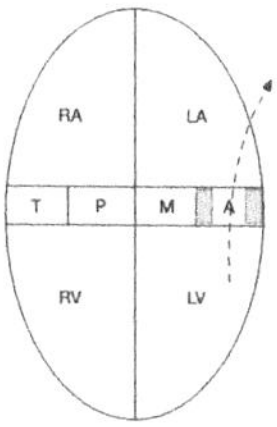

Etiology: calcification (smoking, HTN, HLD, DM), congenital, rheumatic heart Dz, CT Dz, rad, CKD

AMB: CP, syncope, DOE, paresthesia UE, pulsus tardus, Sx HF poor prognostic

ASx mild Dz: echo q3-5y
ASx mod Dz: q1-2y
ASx Sev Dz: q6-12m (gradient >40, vale <1 sqcms)

Sx + Sev Dz, replace, transcath. Aortic valve replacement (TAVR) if depressed EF; 1st do angiogram

Mitral Stenosis

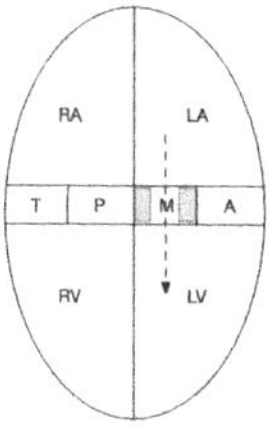

Etiology: rheumatic heart Dz, congenital, SLE, mitral annular calcification d/t aging or amyloidosis

AMB: DOE, AF

CXR: straightening of left heart border

Complications: LA dilation → AF → embolism & HF

If valve < 1.3 sq cms (mild), then do valvuloplasty

Mod-severe, then do valve repair

Use diltiazem of BB to ↑ diastolic filling time

Aortic Regurgitation

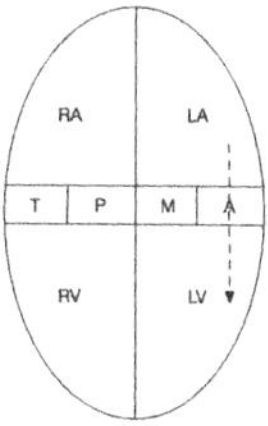

Etiology: RHD, Marfan, CT Dz, Syphilis

AMB: DOE, CP, HF, dizziness, palpitations, DeMusset (bob), Quicken (flush/pallor nails), Traube (pistol shot)

End systolic < 40, End diastolic < 60: echo in 6-12mo

End systolic >50, End diastolic > 65: surgery

Symptomatic w/ EF < 50%: surgery

Mitral Regurgitation

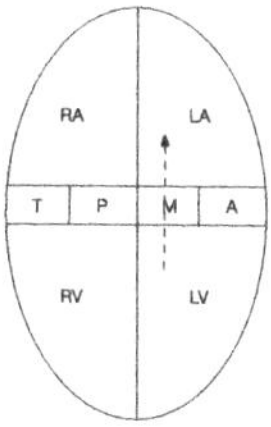

Etiology: A (IE, pap. Muscle, RHD, MI); C (myxomatous, MVP, mitral annular enlargement)

AMB: dysp., orthop., PND, dysphagia, PVC/SVT

↑ End syst/diast measurements +

- LVEF < 60%
- pHTN
- AF
- Symptomatic

→ surgery, repair > replacement (mortality, POD comp.)

Valve Replacement	
Mechanical	**Bioprosthetic**
ASA 81 mg PO qd + Warfarin PO qd w/ goal INR 2.5 – 3.0	ASA 81 mg PO qd + Warfarin w/ goal INR 2.0 – 3.0 x 3 mo

Infective Endocarditis (IE)

Etiology:
- Native valve endocarditis (NVE)
- Prosthetic valve endocarditis (PVE)
- IV drug abuse (IVDA) infective endocarditis
- Nosocomial/Healthcare-associated infective endocarditis
- Fungal endocarditis

Manifestations:
- Fever, low-grade and intermittent (90% pts)
- Murmur (85% pts)
- 1+ classic sign (50% pts)
    - Petechiae
    - **Subungal (splinter) hemorrhages**
    - **Osler nodes** – tender SQ nodules on digits
    - **Janeway lesions** – maculae palms/soles
    - **Roth spots** – retinal hem./small, clear centers

Major Criteria	
Positive Blood Cultures Typical pathogens from at least 2 separate cultures	
Evidence of endocardial involvement by echocardiogram Endocardial vegetation, perivalvular abscess, new partial dehiscence of prosthetic valve, new valvular regurgitation	
Minor Criteria	
Predisposition Heart condition or IVDU	**Fever** $\geq 38^{\circ}C$
Microbiological Evidence Single positive blood culture (except for coagulase-negative Staph or an organism that doesn't cause endocarditis)	**Vascular Phenomena** Arterial emboli, mycotic aneurysm, septic pulmonary infarcts, conjunctival hemorrhages, Janeway lesions
Echocardiographic Findings Consistent with endocarditis, but does not meet major criteria	

Management: Treat HF, O2, empiric Abx (Vancomycin, Piperacillin-tazobactam, Linezolid if AKI/CKD), VTE Prophylaxis

Rheumatic Endocarditis

Inflammatory Dz involving joints, heart, skin, and nervous system. Sequela of group A streptococcal pharyngitis, latent period 18 days.

Jones Criteria (2 major OR 1 major and 2 minor w/ recent GAS infxn):
- J – Joints (Polyarthritis)
- O – Carditis
- N – Nodules
- E – Erythema Migrans
- S – Shaking – Chorea

- Arthralgia
- Prolonged PR interval
- Fever
- Elevated ESR/CRP

Management:
- PCN DOC, cephalosporins if allergic
- Salicylates
- Corticosteroids/digoxin for severe carditis
- Haloperidol for chorea
- Valve replacement/repair

EKG Interpretation & Arrhythmias

1. Identify P-QRS -T waves: Normal Beats, Abnormal Beats
2. Measure PRI, QRS & QT; Measure P to P and R to R for rhythm & rate
3. Identify Rhythm

Bundle Branch Block Normal: QRS Width < 0.11 sec   V1-2 R -VAT< 0.04 sec
V5-6 L -VAT <0.06 sec

Right BBB		**Left BBB**	
V1-2	RSR′	V1-V2	QS or rS, negative complexes
V5-6 & Lead I, aVL	Fat, "Slurred	V5-6 & Lead I, aVL	Notched R wave, no q wave, positive complexes
QRS	>0.12 sec	QRS	Monomorphic, >0.12 sec
Right VAT (V1-2)	Prolonged	Left VAT (V5-6)	Prolonged
ST-T Wave Changes	V1-2	ST-T Wave Changes	I, aVL & V5-6
Right Axis Shift		Left Axis Shift	
		Difficult to recognize MI with LBBB	

Left Anterior Hemiblock
LAD: -30° to -90°
Lead I: qR or R wave
III, ?II, ?aVF: rS
QRS: normal width
Bifascicular Block: RBBB, LAH, LPH

Left Posterior Hemiblock
RAD: +90° to +180°
Lead I: s wave
Lead III: q wave
QRS: normal width
Exclude: RAE and/or RVH, et al. RAD

Atrial Abnormality

Normal P wave: Lead II Sinus P Wave amplitude 2.5 mm and width 0.10 sec
V1-2 Biphasic P wave Positive 1.5 mm amplitude; 0.06s width
Negative 1mm amplitude; 0.04s width

RAE P Wave - P-pulmonale
Lead II/III: Tall, peaked, >2.5 mm
V1: P V1 > P V6

LAE P Wave – P-mitrale
Lead I/II: notched, M shaped, >0.12 sec
Space between humps > 0.04 sec
V1-2: Biphasic, 2nd half P > 0.04 sec

Ventricular Hypertrophy

Normal QRS: Frontal R waves = 5 - 20 mm Precordial S wave or R wave = 7 – 30 mm R > s wave V1-2 rS wave; V5-6 R > s wave

RVH
V1-2: Large R, R:S ratio ≥ 1
Lead I, aVL, V5-6 Deep S, S > r
RAD
RAE
Strain pattern: ST segment depression, downward concavity; T wave inverted

LVH
S (V1 orV2) + R (V5 or V6) ≥ 35 mm
Any precordial lead ≥ 45 mm
R wave I or aVL ≥ 11 – 12 mm
R wave aVF ≥ 20 mm
Strain pattern: ST segment downward concavity; T wave inverted left precordial leads V4-V6

- **Pericarditis**: PR depression, diffuse ST elevation, notching at end of QRS, upward concave ST segments
- **Pericardial Effusion**: ↓amplitude
- **Hypothermia**: Osborn (J) waves
- **Hyperkalemia**: Tall, peaked T waves
- **Hypokalemia**: Flat T waves & prominent U waves
- **Hypercalcemia**: short QT interval
- **Hypocalcemia**: Long QT interval
- **Digoxin**: Scooped ST & inverted T wave
- **Quinidine**: Long QT interval

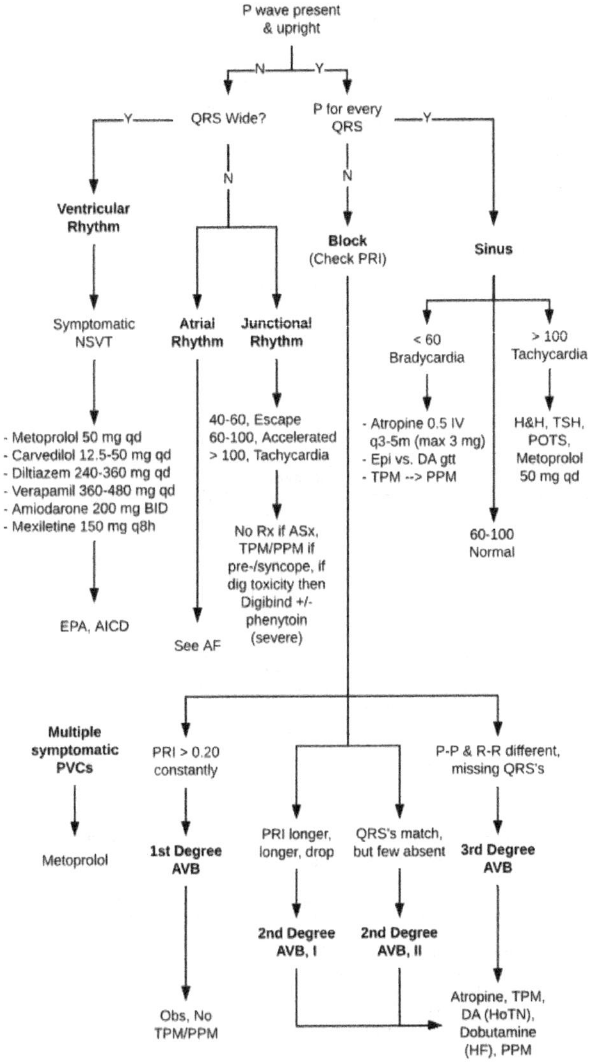

P wave present & upright
N
Y
QRS Wide?
P for every QRS
Y
N
N
Y
Ventricular Rhythm
Block (Check PRI)
Sinus
Symptomatic NSVT
Atrial Rhythm
Junctional Rhythm
< 60 Bradycardia
> 100 Tachycardia
- Metoprolol 50 mg qd
- Carvedilol 12.5-50 mg qd
- Diltiazem 240-360 mg qd
- Verapamil 360-480 mg qd
- Amiodarone 200 mg BID
- Mexiletine 150 mg q8h
40-60, Escape
60-100, Accelerated
> 100, Tachycardia
- Atropine 0.5 IV q3-5m (max 3 mg)
- Epi vs. DA gtt
- TPM --> PPM
H&H, TSH, POTS, Metoprolol 50 mg qd
No Rx if ASx, TPM/PPM if pre-/syncope, if dig toxicity then Digibind +/- phenytoin (severe)
60-100 Normal
EPA, AICD
See AF
Multiple symptomatic PVCs
Metoprolol
PRI > 0.20 constantly
1st Degree AVB
Obs, No TPM/PPM
PRI longer, longer, drop
QRS's match, but few absent
2nd Degree AVB, I
2nd Degree AVB, II
P-P & R-R different, missing QRS's
3rd Degree AVB
Atropine, TPM, DA (HoTN), Dobutamine (HF), PPM

Atrial Fibrillation

Classification:

- **Paroxysmal** – terminates w/in 48h
- **Persistent** – sustained > 7 d or terminated after Rx
- **Permanent** – lasts > 1 yr or cardioversion failed
- **Lone** – age < 60, w/out echo evidence of cardiac Dz

Workup:

- EKG – irregularly irregular rhythm, no P wave
- CXR – cardiomegaly suggesting chronic HTN/LVH
- TTE – LA size, thrombus, valves, LV Fx, pericardium
- K, M – electrolyte induced, predisposition
- TSH/T4 - hyperthyroidism

Etiologies (interference SA-AV):

A	Cardiac	HF, myo/pericarditis, MI, hypertensive crisis, cardiac surgery
C	Pulmonary	PNA, AECOPD, PE, OSA
U	Metabolic	High catecholamines (stress, infxn, post-op, pheo), hyperthyroid
T	Drugs	ETOH, cocaine, amphetamines, caffeine
E	Neuro	SAH, ischemic CVA
CHRONIC		Advanced age, HTN, ischemia, valvular Dz, hyperthyroid, obesity

	Agent	Acute (IV)	Maintenance (PO)	Comments
CCB	Verapamil	5-10 mg over 2 min, repeat q30m	120-360 mg/d in divided doses	- HoTN (Rx w/ Ca gluconate) - May worsen HF - DOC if severe COPD - Can ↑ Dig level
	Diltiazem	0.25 mg/kg over 2 min, repeat after 15 min OR 5-15 mg/h infusion	120-360 mg/d in divided doses	
BB	Metoprolol	5 mg over 2 min, repeat q5min x 3	25-100 mg PO BID or TID	HoTN (Rx w/ glucagon), Mon for HF & bronchospasm; DOC if CAD
	Propranolol	1 mg q2min	80-240 mg/d in divided doses	
Digoxin		0.25 mg q2h up to 1.5 mg	0.125-0.375 mg qd (adjust for CrCl)	Consider if HF or HoTN; poor exertional HR ctrl.
Amiodarone		150 mg bolus over 10 min, then 0.5-1 mg/min x 24h	< 2 wk, 400-800 mg divided until 6-10 g loaded, then 200-400 mg qd > 2 wk, 200-400 mg qd	

	CHA_2DS_2-VASc	Pts	HAS-BLED	Pts
C	CHF/LV systolic dysfunction	1	HTN (uncontrolled)	1
H	HTN (BP > 140/90, or Rx'd)	1	Abnormal renal/liver Fx	1-2
A_2	Age ≥ 75	2	Stroke	1
D	DM	1	Bleed predisposition (Hx)	1
S_2	Prior stroke, TIA, DVT	2	Labile INR	1
V	Vascular Dz (PAD, MI, aortic plaque)	1	Age > 65	1
A	Age 65-74	1	Drugs (e.g., ASA, NSAIDs, clopidogrel, etc.)	1
Sc	Sex category (i.e., female)	1	Drugs (ETOH > 8 drinks/d)	1

> 2, anticoagulate (ASA + clopidogrel, warfarin w/ UFH bridge, dabigatran, apixaban)	One-year bleed risk, >3 Alternative!	
	1 = 3.4% 2 = 4.1% 3 = 5.8%	4 = 8.9% 5 = 9.1% > 5 = >10%

ACLS, Pulse Present

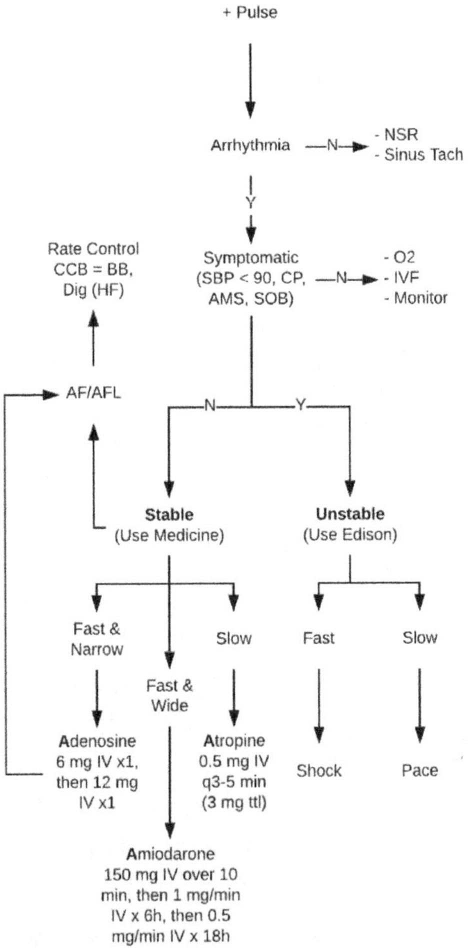

ACLS, Pulse Absent

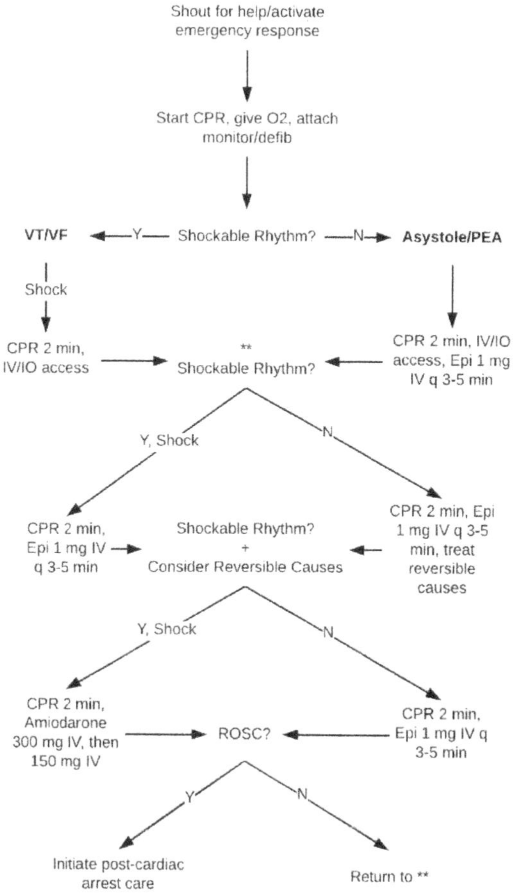

Identifying and Treating the H's & T's

Potential Cause	How to Identify	Treatments
Hypovolemia	Rapid HR and narrow QRS, dry, ↑ BUN/SCr	Infusion of LR or NS
Hypoxemia	Slow HR, SpO2, RR, underlying Dz, trend	Airway management, ventilation
Hydrogen Ion Excess (Acidosis)	Low amplitude QRS, Low HCO3, High PaCO2, gap	Hyperventilation, consider sodium bicarb
Hypokalemia	Flat T waves + U wave	IV magnesium/Potassium
Hyperkalemia	Peaked T waves, wide QRS	CaCl, sodium bicarb, insulin + glucose
Hypothermia	Exposure to cold, hypothyroidism	Gradual re-warming, ?Levothyroxine
Hyperthermia	Anesthesia, antipsychotic, antidepressant	Dantrolene sodium, cyproheptadine

Potential Cause	How to Identify	Treatments
Tension PTX	Slow HR, narrow QRS, dyspnea, US absent pleural sliding or barcode sign	Thoracostomy or needle decompression
Tamponade	Rapid HR, narrow QRS (low amplitude, QRS alternans), US RA collapse + effusion	Pericardiocentesis
Thromboembolism (PE)	Rapid HR, narrow QRS, US RV strain (McConnell's sign)	Fibrinolytics, anticoagulants (heparin gtt), surgical embolectomy
Thrombosis (MI)	ST elevation, abn cardiac biomarkers	Cardiac cath for PCI, heparin gtt

Code Workup: CBC (hemorrhage, dehydration), CMP (BUN/SCr, lytes), Mag, troponin, D-dimer, bedside US

Post-Arrest Care

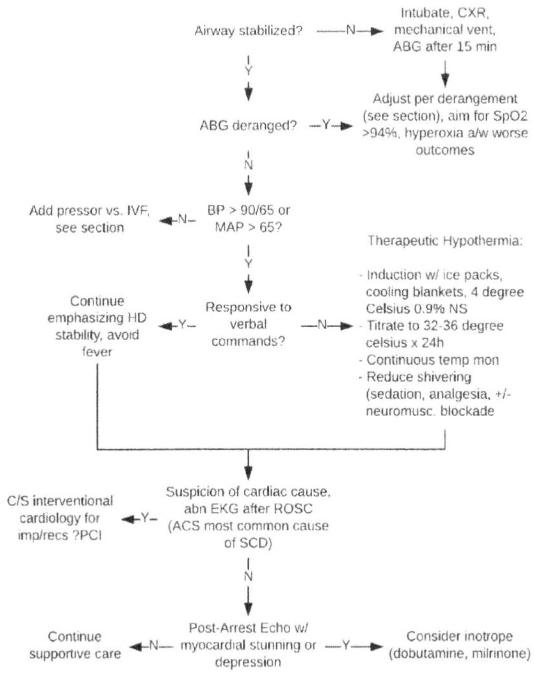

Prognostication

Without Therapeutic Hypothermia	With Therapeutic Hypothermia
Early prognostic indicators via neuro exam @ 72 hrs, delay prognostication in those receiving sedation/paralysis	Early prognostication @ 72 hrs after return to normothermia

Aneurysm

	Thoracic	Abdominal
Symptoms	CP rad to back, Acute AR w/ decrescendo. Murmur, Widened mediastinum	Intrascapular pain
Dx	CT w/ contrast	TEE, CT w/ contrast if unavailable
Surgery		
Asymptomatic	> 6 cm	> 5 cm
Symptomatic	Any size	Any size
Rx	Surgery, then BB + IV nitroprusside	BB + IV nitroprusside, then Surgery

Screening: Anytime smoker 65-75 y/o male, US ONCE in life; NO screening in female

Frequency of Screening:

< 3 cm, q 5 yrs
3.0 – 3.4 cm, q 3 yrs
3.5 – 4.5 cm, annually
4.5 – 5.0 cm, q 6 mo

Peripheral Vascular Disease (PVD)

Risks:

- Arterial: atherosclerosis/HLD, CKD, smoking, DM, obesity
- Venous: DVT, thrombophlebitis, leg trauma, sustained elevation of venous pressure (e.g., HF)

Manifestations:

- Arterial: claudication, neurovascular (pain, pulselessness, pallor, poikilothermia, paresthesia, paralysis), circular ulceration to affected extremity
- Venous: edema w/ prolonged standing, lower extremity cramping at night, trophic changes w/ brown discoloration, irregular shaped ulceration

Diagnosis:

- Arterial Doppler US to eval flow
- Ankle-brachial index (ABI)
- Arteriography definitive
- If ?venous, R/O other causes of edema (HF, CKD, cirrhosis, etc.)

Management:

- Modify risk factors
- Anticoagulation
- Angioplasty, stenting, bypass, tPA catheter, amputation

Gastroenterology

Nutrition

Assessment:

- Albumin < 3.5 g/dL
  - Indicates protein malnutrition
  - Edema occurs when albumin < 2.7 g/dL
- Pre-albumin
  - Earliest indicator of malnutrition
- Hgb < 12 g/dL (female) or < 13.5 g/dL (male)
  - May indicate lack of iron or protein → lack of O2 delivery
- Clinical observations
  - Hair not easily plucked (wiry)
  - Musculature
  - Clear nail beds free of ridges
  - Pink/moist mucous membranes

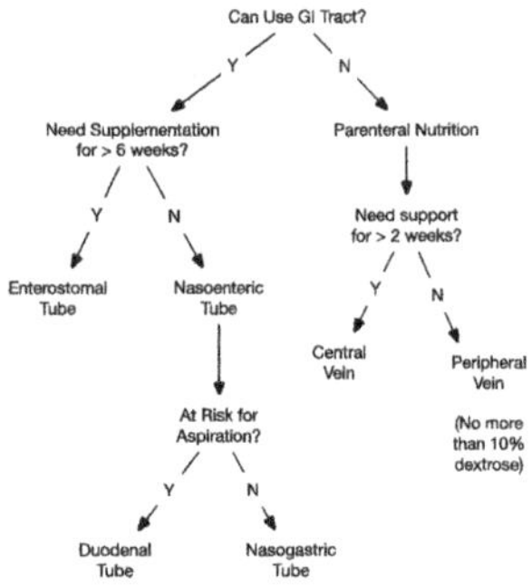

Enteral Complications:

- Aspiration
- Diarrhea
- Emesis
- GIB
- Mechanical obstruction of tube
- Hypernatremia
- Dehydration

Parenteral Complications:

- Pneumothorax
- Hemothorax
- Arterial laceration
- Air emboli
- Catheter thrombosis
- Catheter-associated infxn
- Hyperglycemia
- HHNS

Malnutrition Assessment

	Acute Illness		Chronic Illness		Social/Environmental	
	Mod	Severe	Mod	Severe	Mod	Severe
Energy Intake	< 75% est. req. >7 days	≤ 50% est. req. ≥ 5 days	< 75% est. req. ≥1 mo	≤ 75% est. req. ≥1 mo	< 75% est. req. ≥3 mo	≤ 50% est. req. ≥ 1 mo
Wt Loss	1-2%, 1 wk; 5% 1 mo; 7.5% 3 mo	>2% 1 wk; >5% 1 mo; >7.5% 3 mo	5% 1 mo; 7.5% 3 mo; 10% 6 mo; 20% 1 yr	>5% 1 mo; >7.5% 3 mo; >10% 6 mo; >20% 1 yr	5% 1 mo; 7.5% 3 mo; 10% 6 mo; 20% 1 yr	>5% 1 mo; >7.5% 3 mo; >10% 6 mo; >20% 1 yr
Body Fat	Mild	Mod	Mild	Severe	Mild	Severe
MSK Mass	Mild	Mod	Mild	Severe	Mild	Severe
Fluid	Mild	Mod to severe	Mild	Severe	Mild	Severe
Grip Str.	N/A	Reduced	N/A	Reduced	N/A	Reduced

RUQ Abdominal Pain

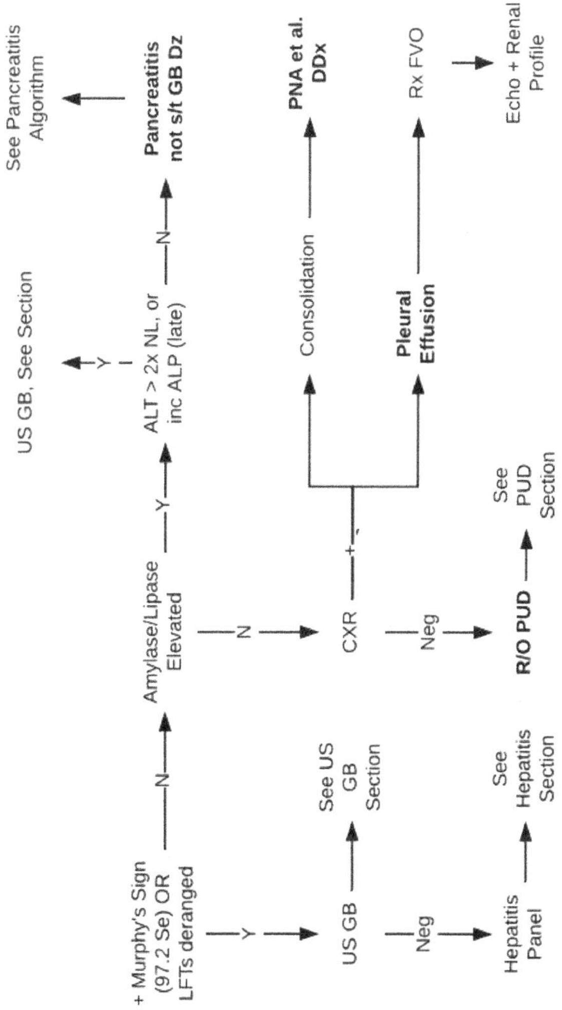

Gallbladder Ultrasound

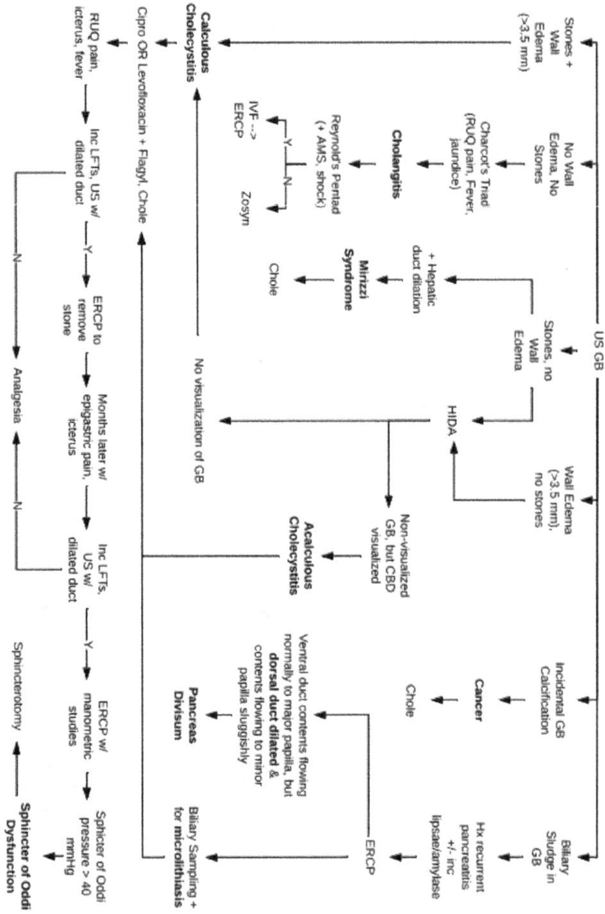

Epigastric Pain

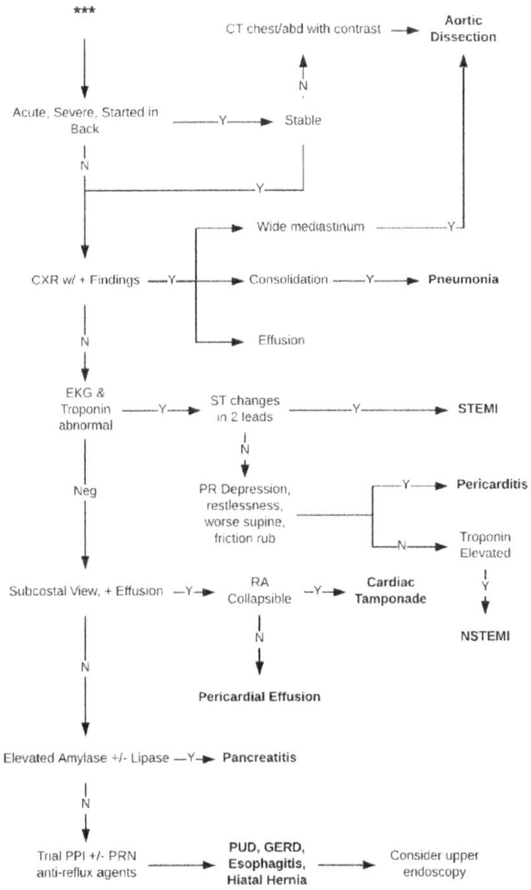

LUQ Pain

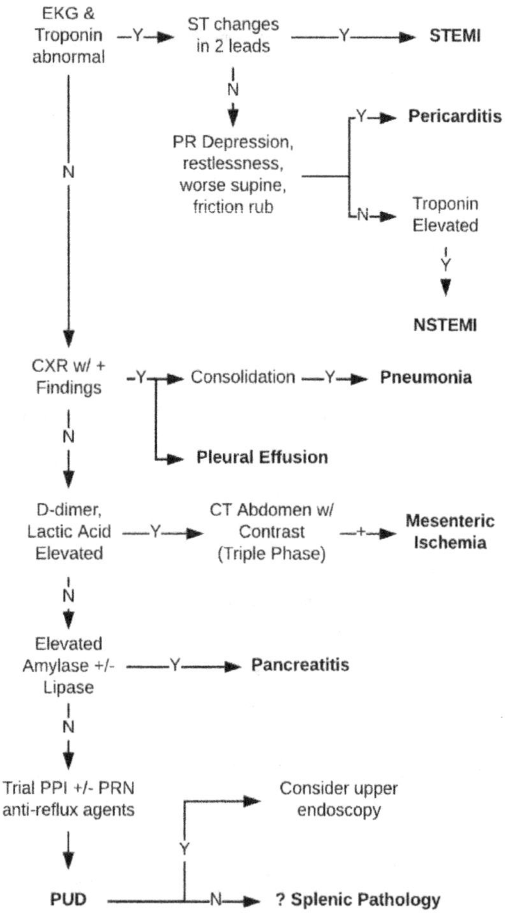
EKG & Troponin abnormal
Y
ST changes in 2 leads
Y
STEMI
N
PR Depression, restlessness, worse supine, friction rub
Y
Pericarditis
N
Troponin Elevated
Y
NSTEMI
N
CXR w/ + Findings
Y
Consolidation
Y
Pneumonia
Pleural Effusion
N
D-dimer, Lactic Acid Elevated
Y
CT Abdomen w/ Contrast (Triple Phase)
+
Mesenteric Ischemia
N
Elevated Amylase +/- Lipase
Y
Pancreatitis
N
Trial PPI +/- PRN anti-reflux agents
PUD
Y
Consider upper endoscopy
N
? Splenic Pathology

Periumbilical Pain

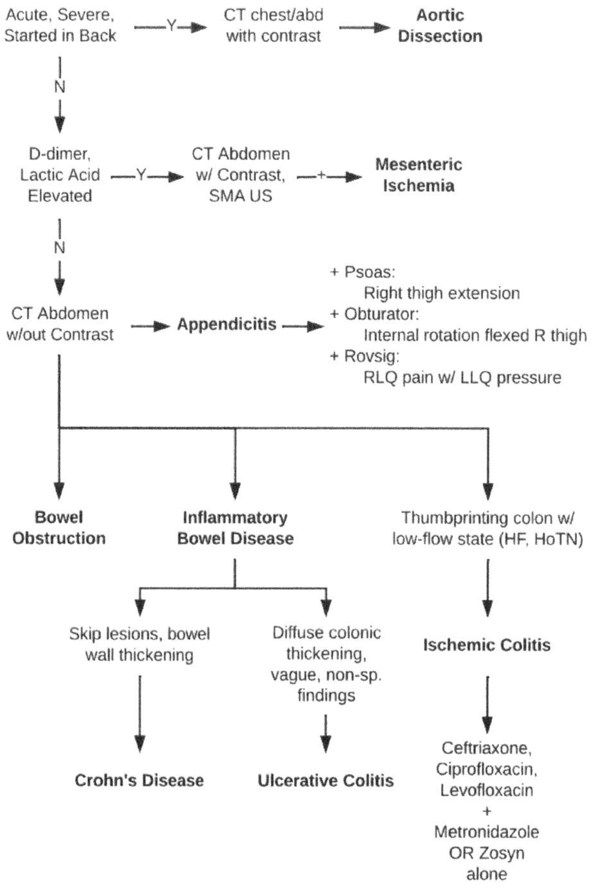

RLQ Pain

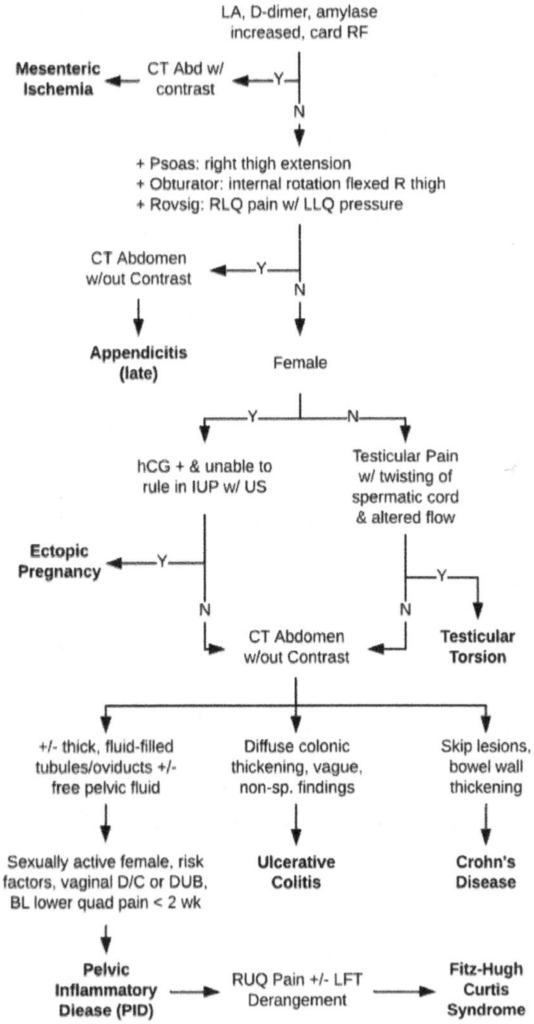
LA, D-dimer, amylase increased, card RF
Y
CT Abd w/ contrast
Mesenteric Ischemia
N
+ Psoas: right thigh extension
+ Obturator: internal rotation flexed R thigh
+ Rovsig: RLQ pain w/ LLQ pressure
Y
CT Abdomen w/out Contrast
Appendicitis (late)
N
Female
Y
N
hCG + & unable to rule in IUP w/ US
Testicular Pain w/ twisting of spermatic cord & altered flow
Y
Ectopic Pregnancy
N
N
Y
Testicular Torsion
CT Abdomen w/out Contrast
+/- thick, fluid-filled tubules/oviducts +/- free pelvic fluid
Diffuse colonic thickening, vague, non-sp. findings
Skip lesions, bowel wall thickening
Sexually active female, risk factors, vaginal D/C or DUB, BL lower quad pain < 2 wk
Ulcerative Colitis
Crohn's Disease
Pelvic Inflammatory Diease (PID)
RUQ Pain +/- LFT Derangement
Fitz-Hugh Curtis Syndrome

Hypogastric Pain

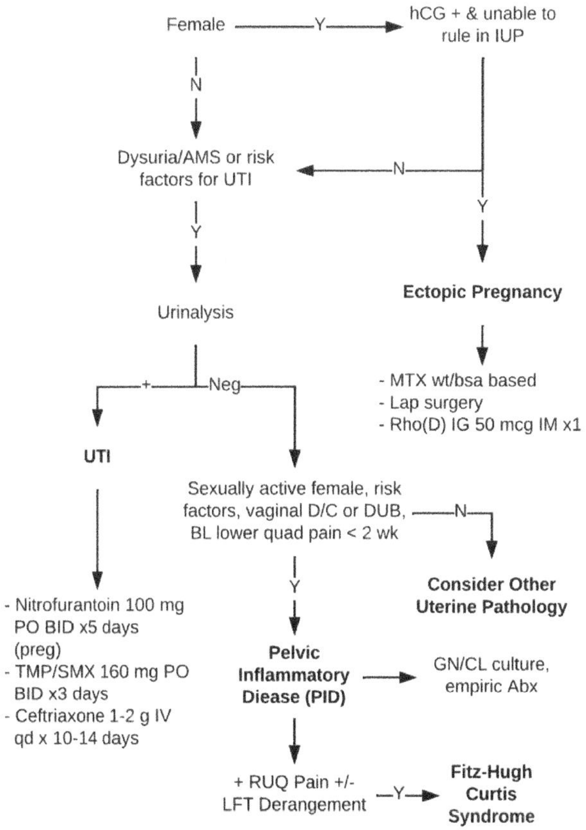

LLQ Pain

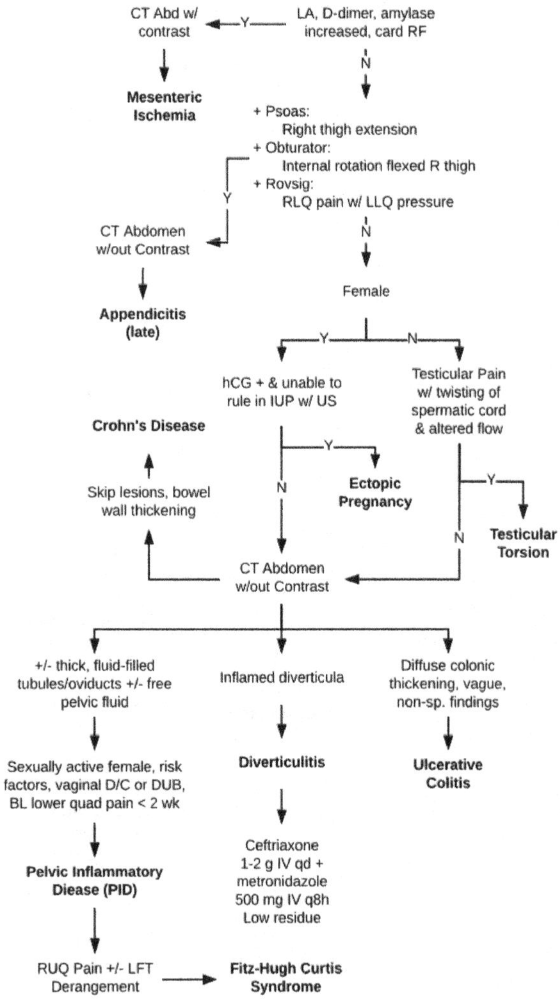
CT Abd w/ contrast
Y
LA, D-dimer, amylase increased, card RF
N
Mesenteric Ischemia
+ Psoas: Right thigh extension
+ Obturator: Internal rotation flexed R thigh
+ Rovsig: RLQ pain w/ LLQ pressure
Y
N
CT Abdomen w/out Contrast
Appendicitis (late)
Female
Y
N
hCG + & unable to rule in IUP w/ US
Testicular Pain w/ twisting of spermatic cord & altered flow
Crohn's Disease
Y
Ectopic Pregnancy
Skip lesions, bowel wall thickening
N
Y
Testicular Torsion
N
CT Abdomen w/out Contrast
+/- thick, fluid-filled tubules/oviducts +/- free pelvic fluid
Inflamed diverticula
Diffuse colonic thickening, vague, non-sp. findings
Sexually active female, risk factors, vaginal D/C or DUB, BL lower quad pain < 2 wk
Diverticulitis
Ulcerative Colitis
Pelvic Inflammatory Diease (PID)
Ceftriaxone 1-2 g IV qd + metronidazole 500 mg IV q8h Low residue
RUQ Pain +/- LFT Derangement
Fitz-Hugh Curtis Syndrome

Abdominal Pain Summary

Right Upper Quadrant (RUQ)	Epigastric	Left Upper Quadrant (LUQ)
- Biliary process (e.g., cholecystitis) - Fitz-Hugh-Curtis Syndrome (PID) - Pancreatitis - PUD - Pleural Process (e.g., effusion) - Pulmonary Process (e.g., PNA) - Hepatitis - Hepatomegaly **CXR, LFTs, US liver/GB, Lipase, Hepatitis Panel, Endoscopy**	- Aortic Aneurysm - Esophageal Pathology (e.g., esophagitis) - Gastric Outlet Obstruction - GERD - Hiatal Hernia - Myocardial Ischemia - Pancreatitis - PUD - Pericardial Process (e.g., Effusion) **EKG, Trops, CXR, Lipase, CT Abd, Endoscopy**	- Mesenteric Ischemia - Myocardial Ischemia - Pancreatitis - PUD - Pleural Process (e.g., Effusion) - Pulmonary Process (e.g., PNA) - Splenic Process (e.g., Splenomegaly) **EKG, Trops, CXR, Lipase, CXR, US of spleen, Endoscopy**
Right Flank	**Periumbilical**	**Left Flank**
- Biliary Process (R only) - Herpes Zoster - Nephrolithiasis - Painful Rib Syndrome - Renal Process (e.g., Infarct, pyelo) - Ureteral Obstruction **BUN/SCr, UA/Cx, LFTs, US GB**	- Aortic Aneurysm - Appendicitis (early) - Bowel Obstruction - Colitis - Inflammatory Bowel Dz - Mesenteric Ischemia **US/CT Abd, US SMA**	- Splenic Process (L only) - Herpes Zoster - Nephrolithiasis - Painful Rib Syndrome - Renal Process (e.g., Infarct, pyelo) - Ureteral Obstruction **BUN/SCr, UA, Foley, US Spleen**
Right Lower Quadrant (RLQ)	**Hypogastric**	**Left Lower Quadrant (LLQ)**
- Ectopic Pregnancy - Pelvic Inflammatory Disease (PID) - Hernia - Hip Joint Pathology - Inflammtory Bowel Dz - Mesenteric Adenitis - Mesenteric Ischemia - Terminal Ileitis - Torsion (testicular, adnexal) - Appendicitis (late) **Abd US/CT, Testicular exam, US SMA, Pregnancy Test, ?GN/CL**	- Bladder Process (e.g., Urinary Retention, UTI) - Ectopic Pregnancy - Pelvic Inflammatory Disease (PID) - Uterine Pathology **US Abd, UA/Cx, BUN/SCr, Pregnancy Test, ?GN/CL**	- Colitis - Diverticulitis - Ectopic Pregnancy - Pelvic Inflammatory Disease (PID) - Hernia - Hip Joint Pathology - Inflammatory Bowel Dz - Torsion (testicular, adnexal) **US/CT Abd, Pregnancy Test, ?GN/CL, Testicular Exam**

Nausea/Vomiting

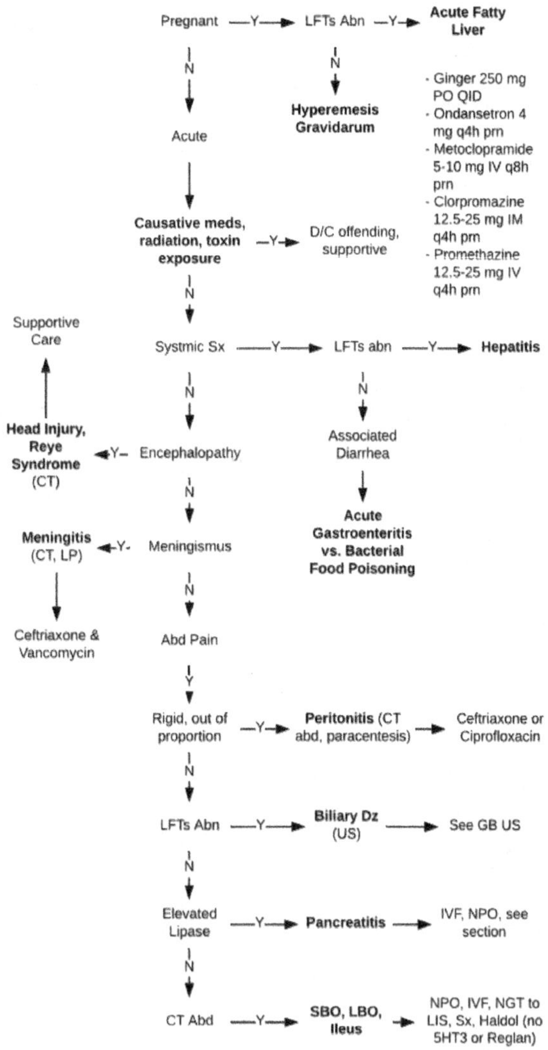

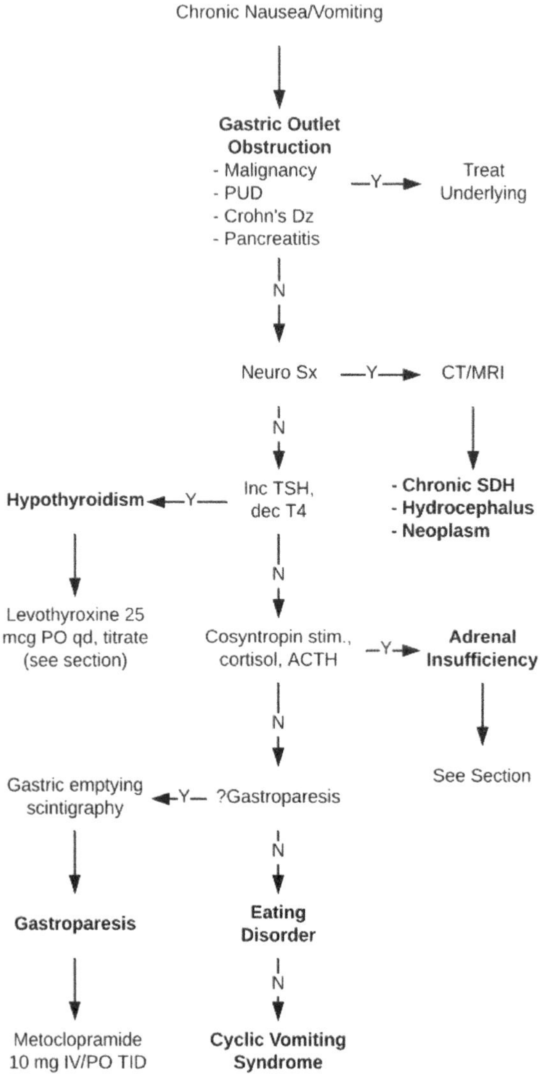
Chronic Nausea/Vomiting
Gastric Outlet Obstruction
- Malignancy
- PUD
- Crohn's Dz
- Pancreatitis
Y
Treat Underlying
N
Neuro Sx
Y
CT/MRI
- Chronic SDH
- Hydrocephalus
- Neoplasm
N
Inc TSH, dec T4
Y
Hypothyroidism
Levothyroxine 25 mcg PO qd, titrate (see section)
N
Cosyntropin stim., cortisol, ACTH
Y
Adrenal Insufficiency
See Section
N
?Gastroparesis
Y
Gastric emptying scintigraphy
Gastroparesis
Metoclopramide 10 mg IV/PO TID
N
Eating Disorder
N
Cyclic Vomiting Syndrome

Acute Diarrhea

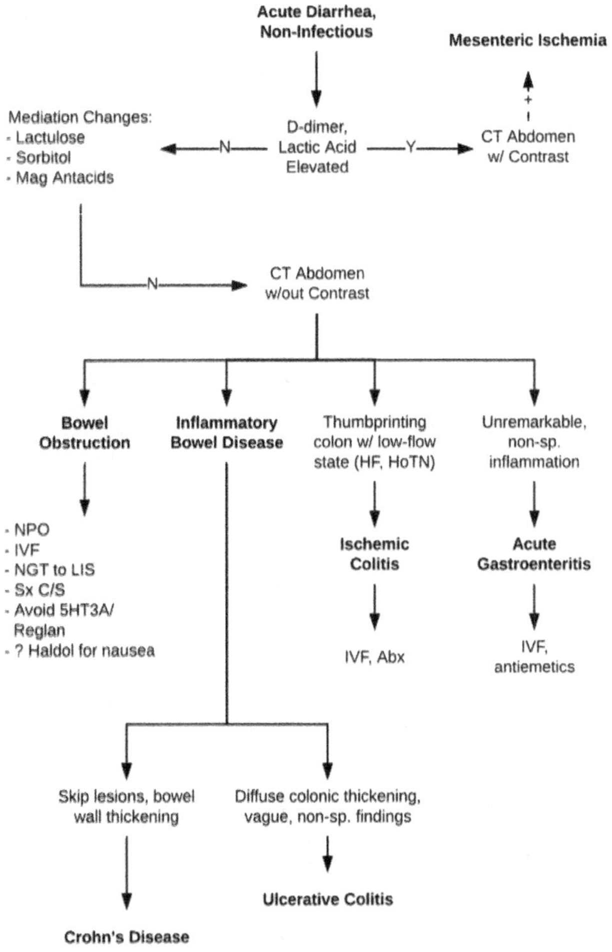

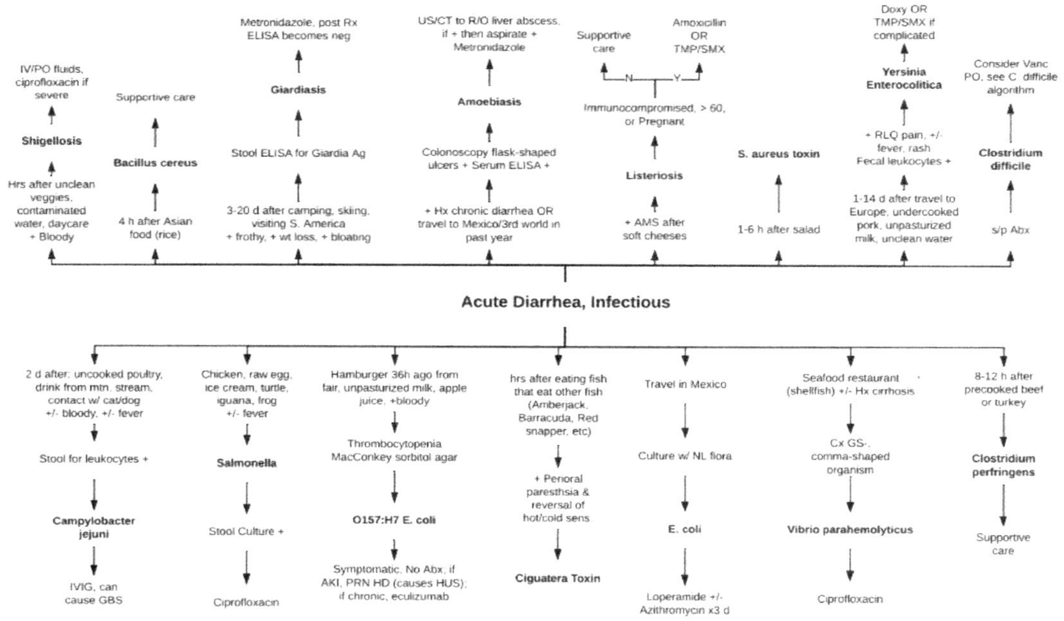

Acute Diarrhea, Infectious
Hrs after unclean veggies, contaminated water, daycare + Bloody
Shigellosis
IV/PO fluids, ciprofloxacin if severe
4 h after Asian food (rice)
Bacillus cereus
Supportive care
3-20 d after camping, skiing, visiting S. America + frothy, + wt loss, + bloating
Stool ELISA for Giardia Ag
Giardiasis
Metronidazole, post Rx ELISA becomes neg
+ Hx chronic diarrhea OR travel to Mexico/3rd world in past year
Colonoscopy flask-shaped ulcers + Serum ELISA +
Amoebiasis
US/CT to R/O liver abscess, if + then aspirate + Metronidazole
+ AMS after soft cheeses
Listeriosis
Immunocompromised, > 60, or Pregnant
N
Y
Supportive care
Amoxicillin OR TMP/SMX
1-6 h after salad
S. aureus toxin
1-14 d after travel to Europe, undercooked pork, unpasturized milk, unclean water
+ RLQ pain, +/- fever, rash Fecal leukocytes +
Yersinia Enterocolitica
Doxy OR TMP/SMX if complicated
s/p Abx
Clostridium difficile
Consider Vanc PO, see C. difficile algorithm
2 d after: uncooked poultry, drink from mtn. stream, contact w/ cat/dog +/- bloody, +/- fever
Stool for leukocytes +
Campylobacter jejuni
IVIG, can cause GBS
Chicken, raw egg, ice cream, turtle, iguana, frog +/- fever
Salmonella
Stool Culture +
Ciprofloxacin
Hamburger 36h ago from fair, unpasturized milk, apple juice, +bloody
Thrombocytopenia MacConkey sorbitol agar
O157:H7 E. coli
Symptomatic, No Abx; if AKI, PRN HD (causes HUS); if chronic, eculizumab
hrs after eating fish that eat other fish (Amberjack, Barracuda, Red snapper, etc)
+ Perioral paresthsia & reversal of hot/cold sens
Ciguatera Toxin
Travel in Mexico
Culture w/ NL flora
E. coli
Loperamide +/- Azithromycin x3 d
Seafood restaurant (shellfish) +/- Hx cirrhosis
Cx GS-, comma-shaped organism
Vibrio parahemolyticus
Ciprofloxacin
8-12 h after precooked beef or turkey
Clostridium perfringens
Supportive care

Chronic Diarrhea

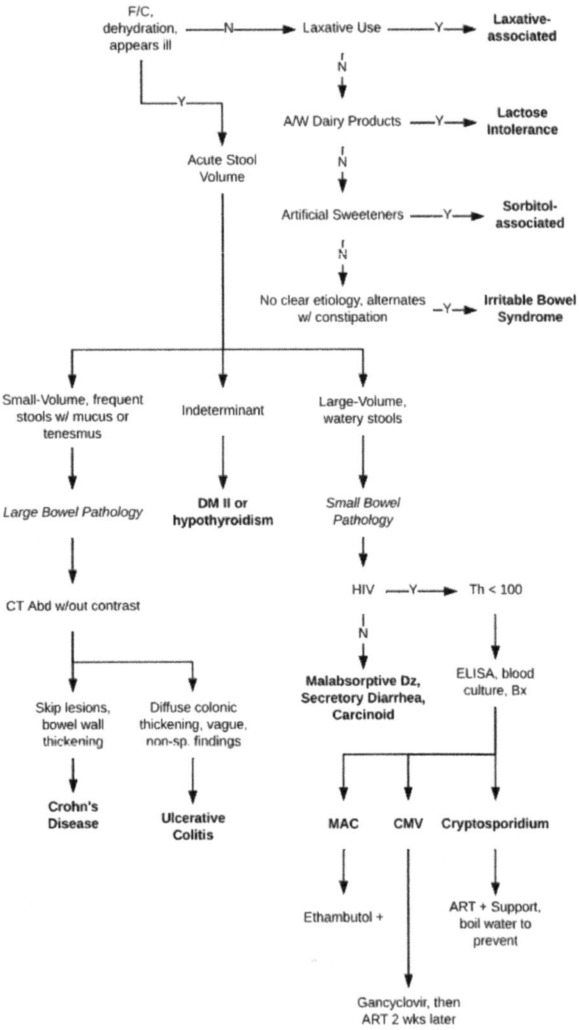

C. Difficile

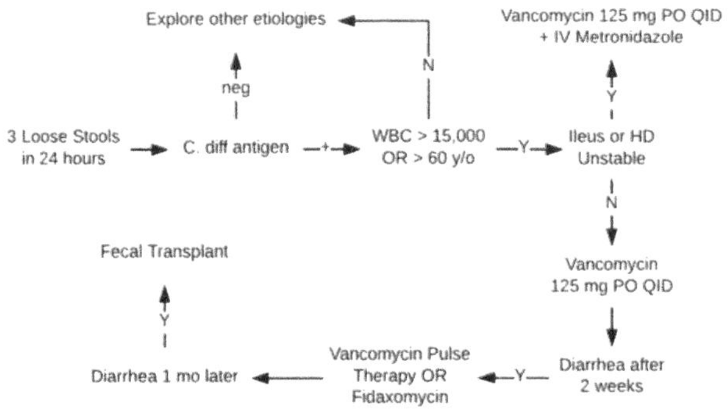

Odynophagia

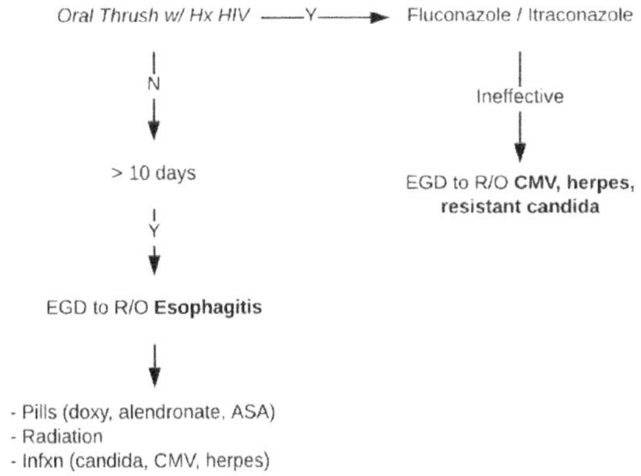

Dysphagia

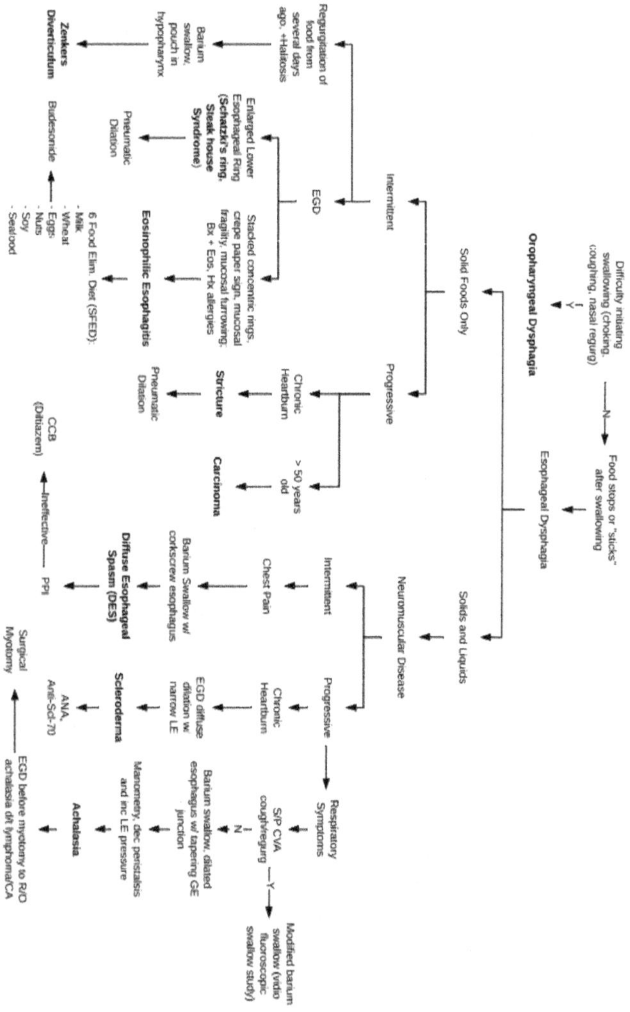

Difficulty initiating swallowing (choking, coughing, nasal regurg)
Y
Oropharyngeal Dysphagia
N
Food stops or "sticks" after swallowing
Esophageal Dysphagia
Solid Foods Only
Intermittent
EGD
Regurgitation of food from several days ago. +Halitosis
Barium swallow, pouch in hypopharynx
Zenkers Diverticulum
Enlarged Lower Esophageal Ring (Schatzki's ring, Steak house Syndrome)
Pneumatic Dilation
Stacked concentric rings, crepe paper sign, mucosal fragility, mucosal furrowing. Bx + Eos, Hx allergies
Eosinophilic Esophagitis
6 Food Elim. Diet (SFED):
- Milk
- Wheat
- Eggs
- Nuts
- Soy
- Seafood
Budesonide
Progressive
Chronic Heartburn
Stricture
Pneumatic Dilation
> 50 years old
Carcinoma
Solids and Liquids
Neuromuscular Disease
Intermittent
Chest Pain
Barium Swallow w/ corkscrew esophagus
Diffuse Esophageal Spasm (DES)
PPI
Ineffective
CCB (Diltiazem)
Progressive
Chronic Heartburn
EGD diffuse dilation w/ narrow LE
Scleroderma
ANA, Anti-Scl-70
Respiratory Symptoms
S/P CVA cough/regurg
Y
Modified barium swallow (video fluoroscopic swallow study)
N
Barium swallow, dilated esophagus w/ tapering GE junction
Manometry, dec peristalsis and inc LE pressure
Achalasia
EGD before myotomy to R/O achalasia d/t lymphoma/CA
Surgical Myotomy

Constipation

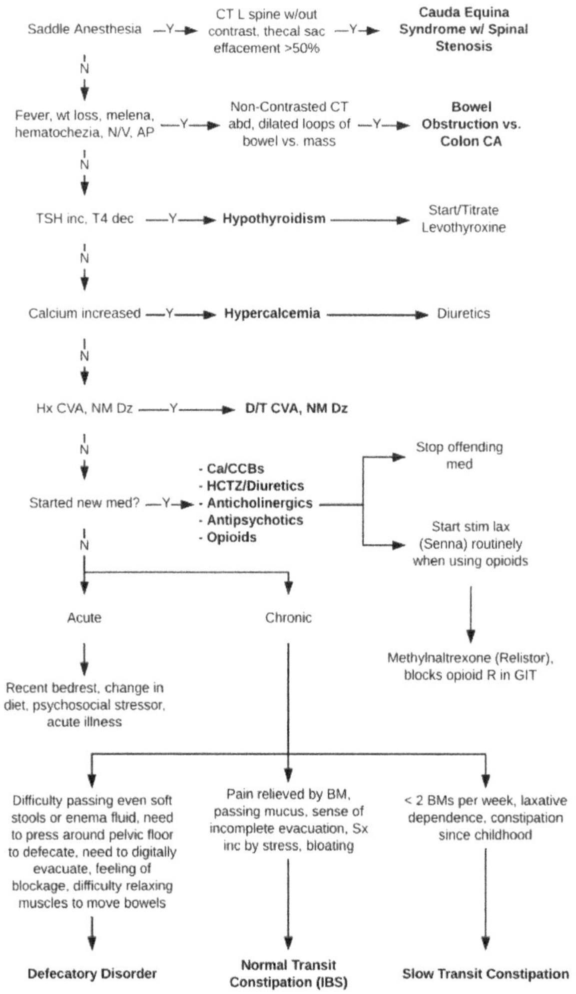

Hematochezia

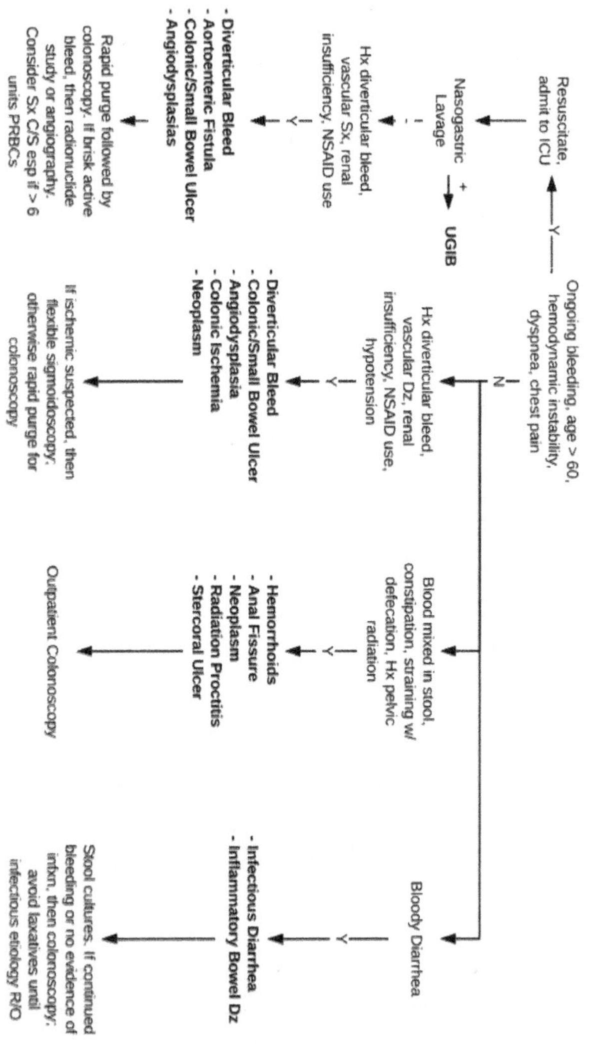

Hematemesis

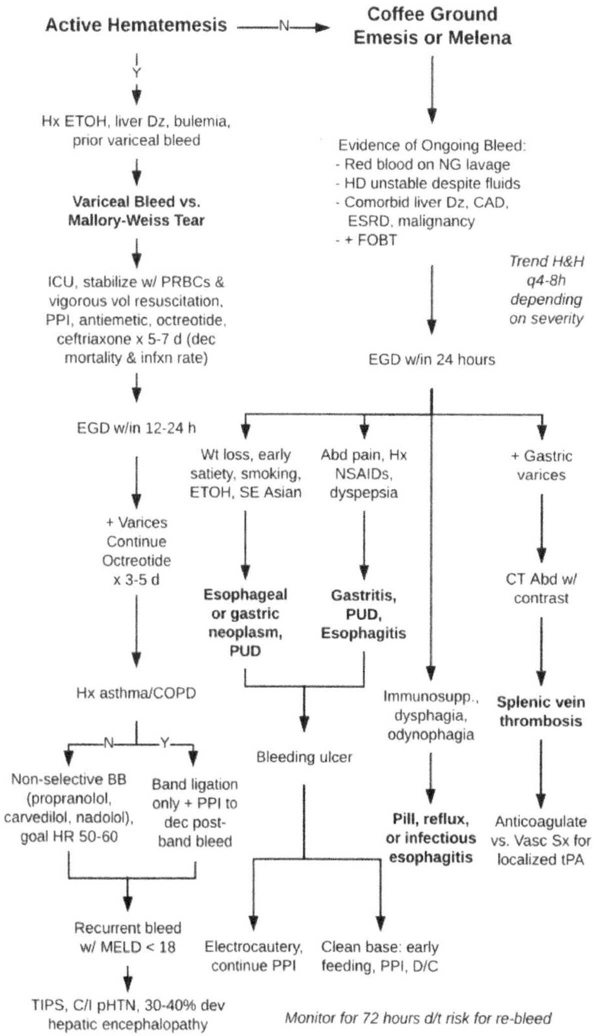

Dyspepsia

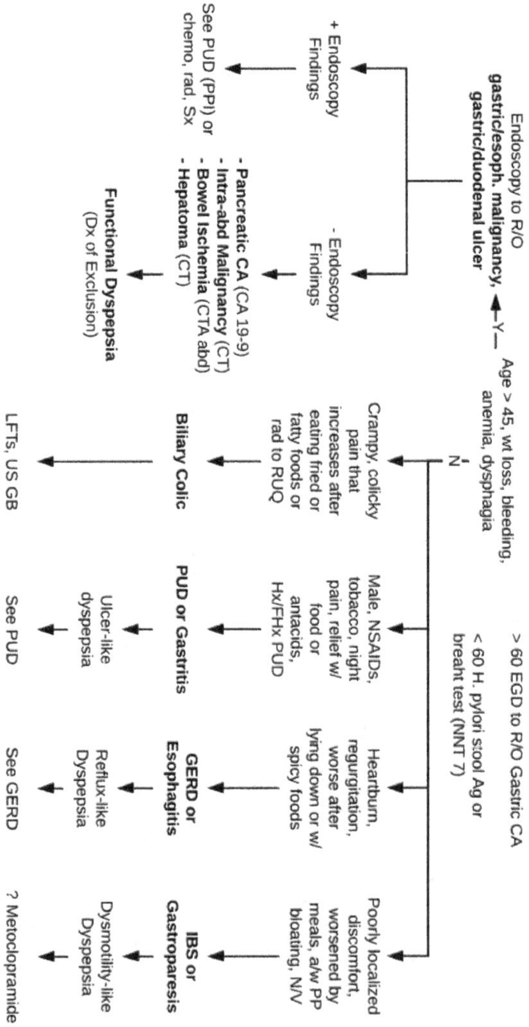
Endoscopy to R/O
gastric/esoph. malignancy,
gastric/duodenal ulcer
Y
Age > 45, wt loss, bleeding, anemia, dysphagia
N
> 60 EGD to R/O Gastric CA
< 60 H. pylori stool Ag or breaht test (NNT 7)
+ Endoscopy Findings
See PUD (PPI) or chemo, rad, Sx
- Endoscopy Findings
- Pancreatic CA (CA 19-9)
- Intra-abd Malignancy (CT)
- Bowel Ischemia (CTA abd)
- Hepatoma (CT)
Functional Dyspepsia
(Dx of Exclusion)
Crampy, colicky pain that increases after eating fried or fatty foods or rad to RUQ
Biliary Colic
LFTs, US GB
Male, NSAIDs, tobacco, night pain, relief w/ food or antacids, Hx/FHx PUD
PUD or Gastritis
Ulcer-like dyspepsia
See PUD
Heartburn, regurgitation, worse after lying down or w/ spicy foods
GERD or Esophagitis
Reflux-like Dyspepsia
See GERD
Poorly localized discomfort, worsened by meals, a/w PP bloating, N/V
IBS or Gastroparesis
Dysmotility-like Dyspepsia
? Metoclopramide

Liver Function Analysis

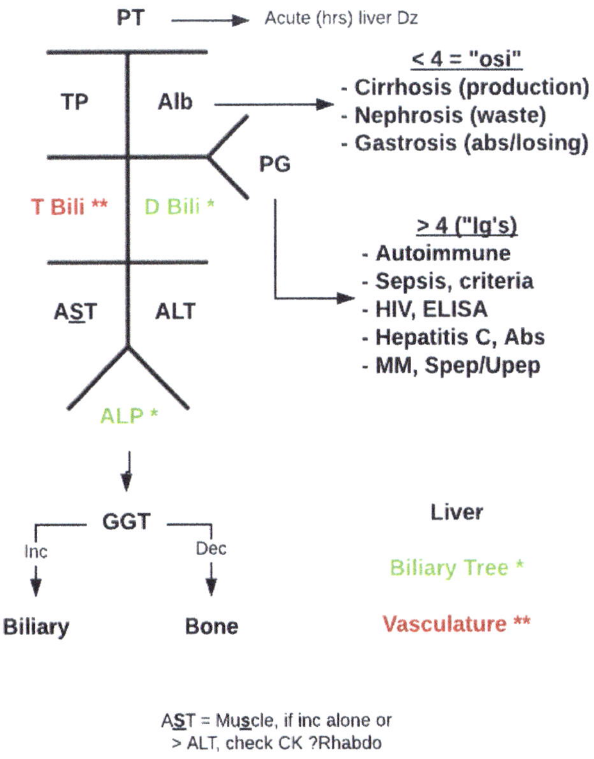

Maddrey's Discriminant Function for Alcoholic Hepatitis:

4.6 (Pt's PT – Control PT) + T. Bili; > 32 suggests poor prognosis, consider steroids

Liver Enzymes in 1000's

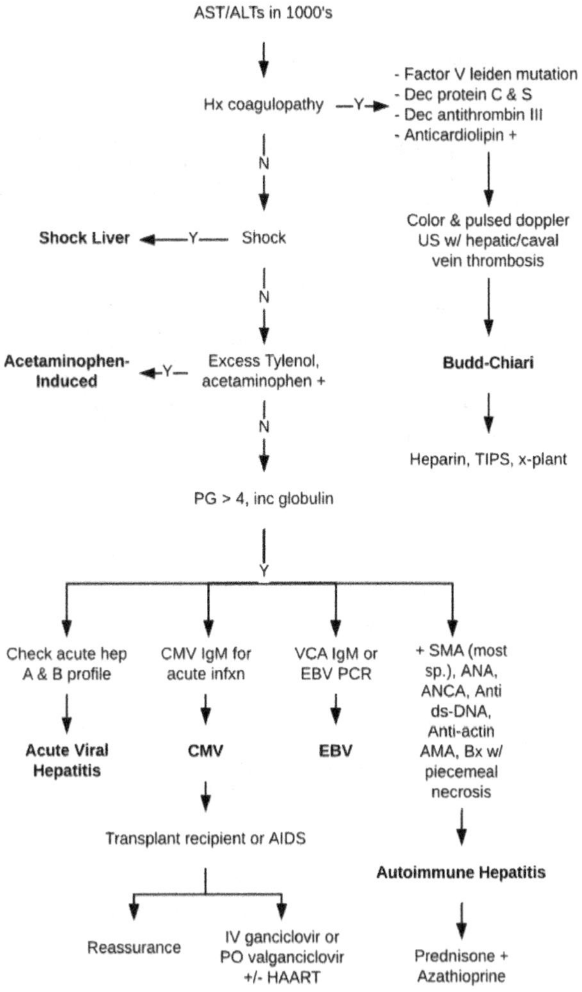

Jaundice

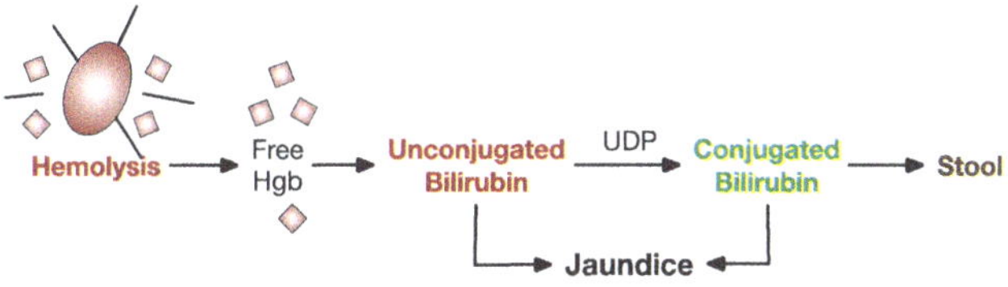

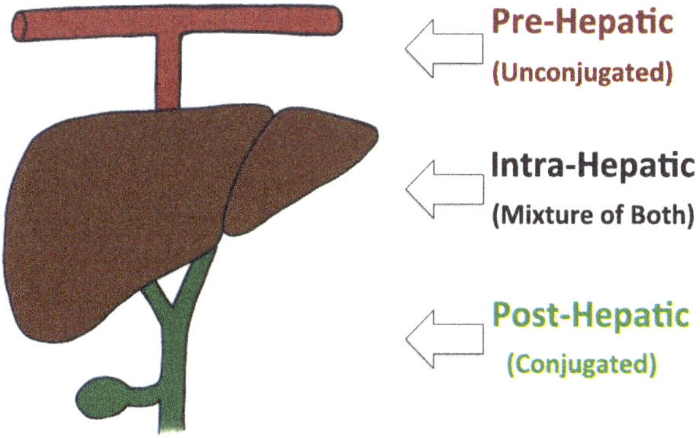

Pre-Hepatic
(Unconjugated)

- Hemolysis
- Hematoma

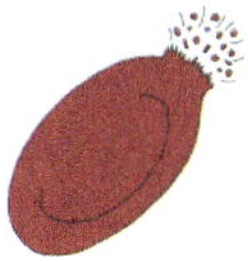

Intra-Hepatic
(Mixture of Both)

- Unconjugated
  - Criggler-Najar
  - Gilbert's
- Conjugated
  - Dubin-Johnson
  - Roter syndrome
- Cirrhosis
- Hepatitis

Post-Hepatic
(Conjugated)

- Painful
  - Gallstones
- Painless
  - Cancer
  - Strictures

Anorectal Pain

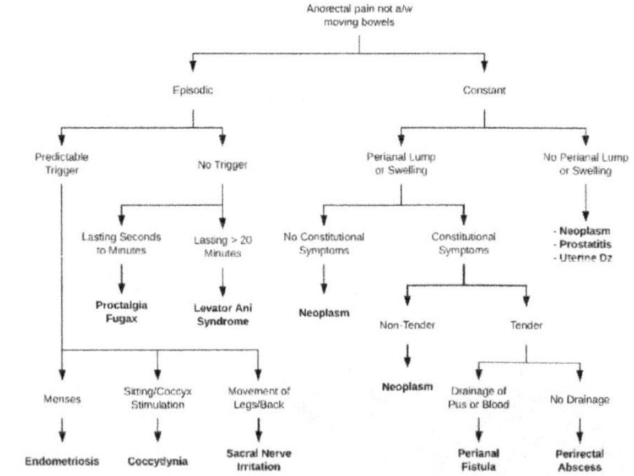

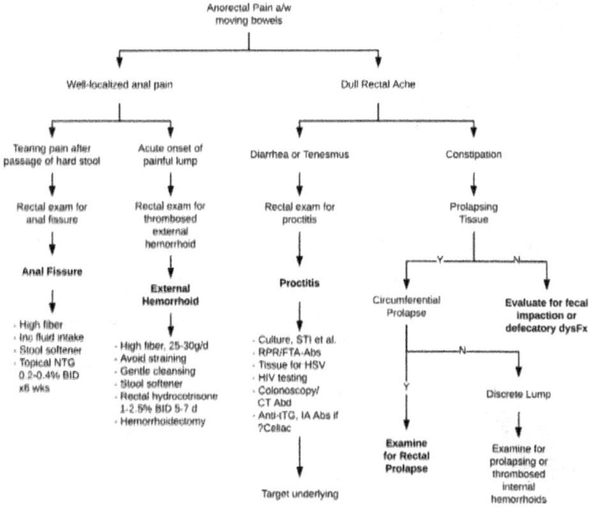

Gastroesophageal Reflux Disease (GERD)

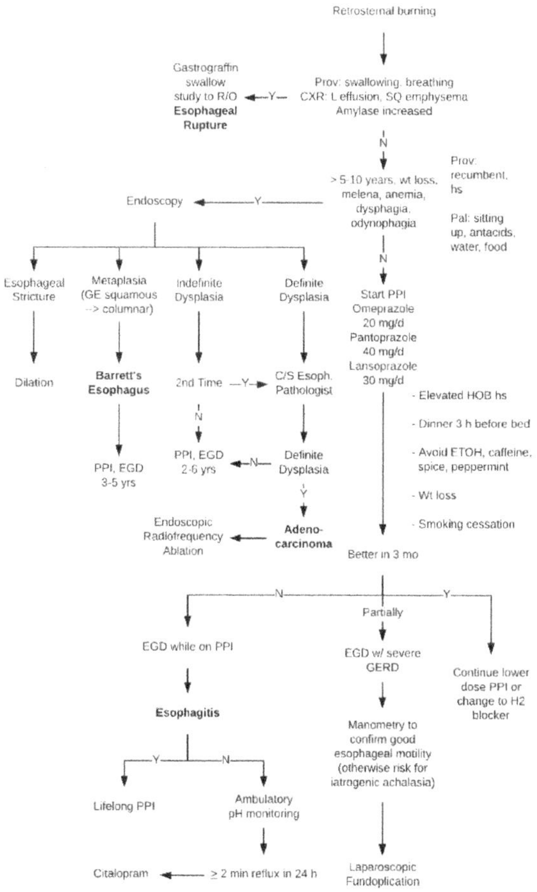

Peptic Ulcer Disease

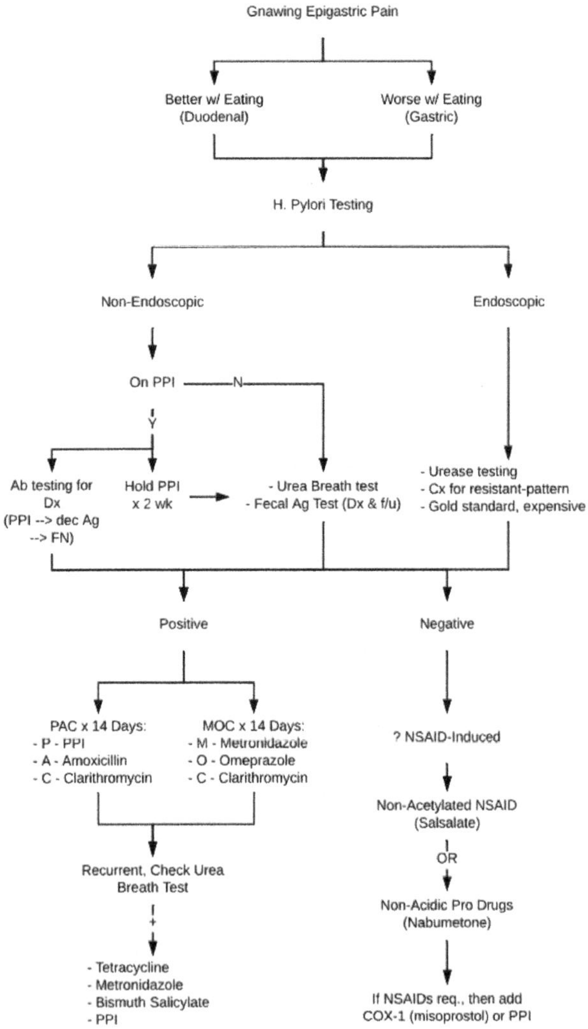

Pancreatitis

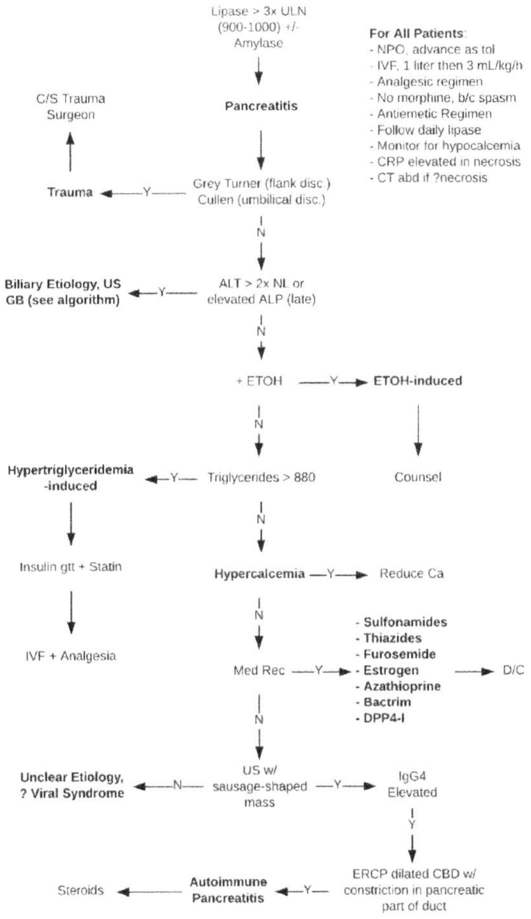

Asymptomatic Pancreatic Cyst

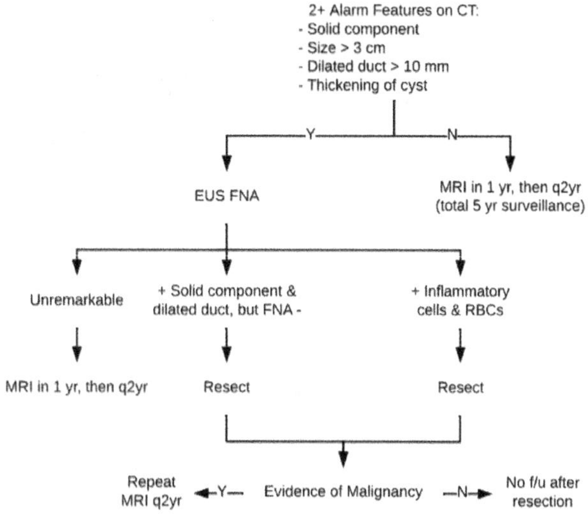

Complications of Pancreatitis

Time Frame	Problem	Findings/Data	Management
Anytime	Splenic vein thrombosis	CT Abdomen w/ contrast	Anticoagulation
4-6 week	Abscess	Soap bubble sign Gram stain of aspirate	Antibiotics, drain tube; if cntd. fever @ 72h, open drain
1-4 weeks	Pseudocyst	> 4 cm may not resolve Comp: pseudoaneurysm, hemorrhage, rupture, fistula	Drainage for symptoms
< 2 weeks	Pancreatic Necrosis	Spiral CT/CT w contrast Comp: MODS	Aggressive fluid 12-24h; Abx vs. CT-guided aspiration if infxn
2 days	Fluid collections, pleual effusion	CXR	Continue aggressive IVF

Cirrhosis

Acute on chronic liver failure: acute decompensation (ascites, encephalopathy, variceal bleed, ↑ INR, jaundice, ↑ bilirubin) + 1 or more extrahepatic organ failure (CLIF-C ACLF Score for ICU 28-day mortality)

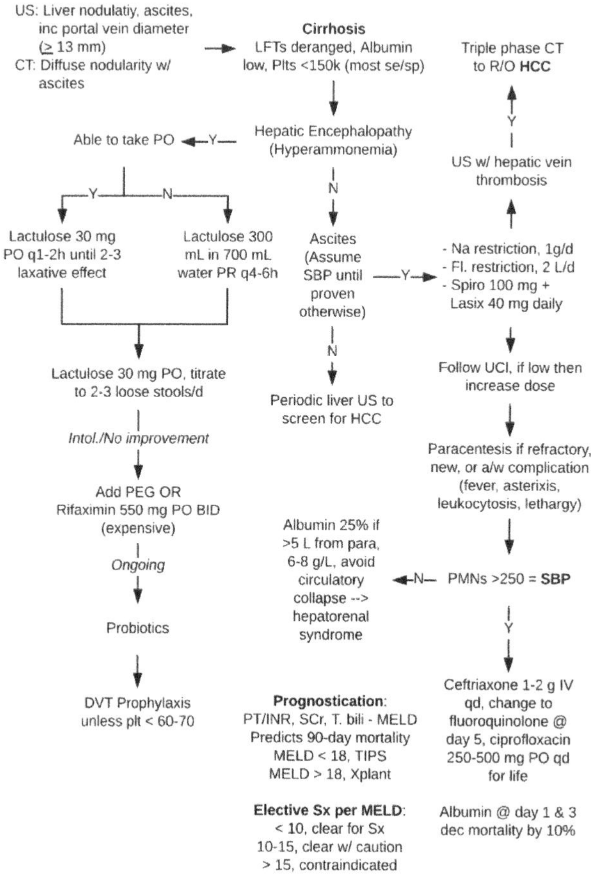

Hepatitis Antibodies

	Route	Acute	Chronic = CA risk	RNA vs. DNA	Vax	Serology
Hep A	Fecal-oral	Y	N	RNA	Y	IgM = IMMediate/Infected IgG = Good = Immune
Hep B	Blood IVDU Sex	Y	Y	DNA	Y	HB_SAg = Infxn HBCAg = Infectious IgM HB_SAg = Early Infxn IgG HB_SAg = Immune IgG HB_CAg = Imm. Exposure
Hep C	Blood IVDU Sex	N	Y	RNA	N	Ab + HCV RNA + = Infected Ab – HCV RNA + = Acute Ab + HCV RNA - = Treated
Hep D	Need HBV	N	Y	DNA	N	Anti-delta antibodies

Liver Transplant

Indications	Contraindications	Relative Contraindications
Cirrhosis w/ decompensation: - Ascites - Variceal bleed - Hepatic encephalopathy Biochemical decompensation: - ↑ SCr - ↑ T. bili - ↑ PT/INR	- Active ETOH - Active illicit use - Extrahepatic CA - Unresolved sepsis or fungemia	- Active HIV or hep C - Hep B w/ e Ag + (Rx for hep B before transplant OR if urgent transplant and give HBIG)

Ascitic Fluid DDx

Albumin	Protein	Condition
Low	High	RHF, hepatic vein thrombosis
Low	Low	Cirrhosis, liver failure, portal vein thrombosis
High	Low	Nephrotic syndrome
High	High	Pancreatitis, peritoneal carcinomatosis, TB
Albumin LOW = portal/hepatic, albumin HIGH = non-portal		

SAAG > 1.1 = Cirrhosis

SAAG < 1.1 = Extrahepatic
(Infxn, peritoneal carcinomatosis, malignancy, renal disease, pancreatitis)

Cirrhosis Etiology

Condition	Risk/History	LFTs	Tests	Management
ETOH Hepatitis	+ ETOH use	AST:ALT 2:1, not >350	BAC, Bx: necrosis of hepatocytes w/ inflammatory Cells	Steroids if no GIB/SBP, otherwise pentoxifylline
Hepatitis A, B	Travel, Sex, IVDU	AST & ALT 100-1000	Hepatitis Profile	Vaccine to prevent
Hepatitis C	IVDU, Sex	AST & ALT 100's	Hepatitis Profile	Ledipasvir/sofosbuvir
NASH	Obese, DM, HLD, OSA, OHS	AST:ALT 1:2-3	Bx: fatty changes w/ some fibrosis	Statin, vitamin E, RF reduction
Hemo-chromatosis	Anemia	Mildly deranged LFTs	↑ Fe & ferritin; Bx: Fe deposition	Chelation
Drug-Induced Hepatitis	Am/Clav,Bactrim, INH, chlorprom., erythromycin, amio, steroids, tetracycline, Reye's syndrome (ASA + flu), methyldopa, trazodone, Macrobid, phenytoin, Tylenol	LFTs in 1000's if a/w acetaminophen	Acetaminophen level	Stop offending agent
Heart Failure	JVD, BLE edema	Mildly elevated LFTs	Echo, BNP	Diurese, ACEI, BB
CMV	HIV	AST/ALT 1000's	CMV IgM	HARRT
EBV	HIV	AST/ALT 1000's	VCA IgM or EBV PCR	HARRT
Autoimmune Hepatitis	Comorbid autoimmune Dz, young, female, arthralgia, rash, icterus	AST & ALT 5-10x ULN	PG > 4, ↑ globulin, + ASMA (most sp.), coombs+	Prednisone + Azathioprine
Wilson's Disease	Young, chronic hepatitis, neuro, hemolytic anemia Kayser-Fleischner rings	AST:ALT > 2, < 2000, ALP < 40, T. bili < 4	↑ urine copper, ↓ serum ceruloplasmin Bx: copper dep.	Chelate: penicillamine + pyridoxine or trientine; liver x-plant
Alpha-1 anti-trypsin Deficiency	Comorbid COPD, FH COPD, non-smoker	Mildly elevated LFTs	↓ AAT	AAT replacement therapy
Budd-Chiari	Coagulopathy Hx	ALT 1000's	Factor V Leiden mutation, ↓protein C & S, ↓ antithrombin III, + anticardiolipin, color & pulse doppler w/ hepatic & caval vein thrombosis	Transplant, Rx cirrhosis, thrombolysis vs. anticoagulation, angio/stent/TIPS
Primary Biliary Cirrhosis	Pruritus @ night, Xanthomas	AST & ALT 2-3x ULN, ALP 1000's	+ AMA, Bx: granulomas /lymphocytic destruction of bile ducts	Early: ursodeoxy-cholate (delays) Late: Liver x-plant
Primary Sclerosing Cholangitis	Hx UC, young, jaundice	AST & ALT NL, ALP ↑	- AMA, Bx: mild inflam. w/ concentric fibrosis around bile ducts (ERCP, MRCP)	Liver transplant, fat-soluble vitamin suppl., avoid infxn, check for IBD
HELLP	Pregnant w/ Hx pre-/ eclampsia	AST & ALT 2-3x ULN	+ Schistocytes, plt ↓, PT NL	Control BP
Acute Fatty Liver of Pregnancy	Pregnant	AST & ALT 2-3 x ULN, ↑ D. bili	+ Schistocytes, plt ↓, PT ↑	Wt loss, diet modification, Rx cirrhosis
Leptospirosis	Sewage, swimming	AST & ALT 1-2x ULN, D. bili 10-50x ULN	Blood, urine, CSF culture + for Leptosporia	Doxycycline, PCN, Erythromycin

Inflammatory Bowel Disease

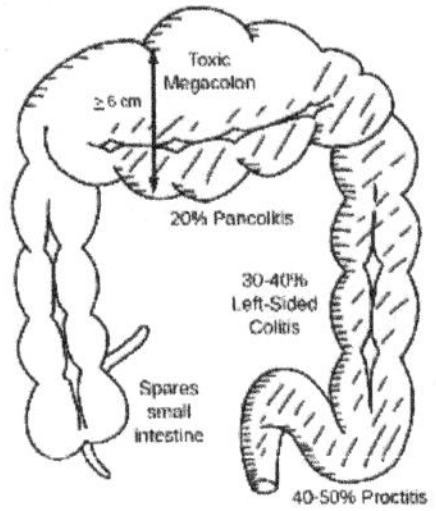

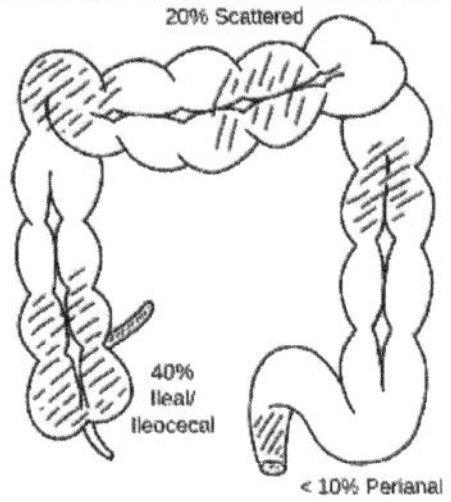

	Ulcerative Colitis (UC)	**Crohn's Disease (CD)**
Pres	- Young, otherwise healthy - Just quit smoking - Often ≥ 6 months - Hematochezia - Abd pain - Diarrhea	- Young, otherwise healthy - Smoking worsens - Often ≥ 6 months - Right lower quad mass - Abd pain - Diarrhea
Extra-Colonic	Mirror: E. nodosum, peripheral arthritis, pyoderma gangrenosum No Mirror: Sacroiliitis, primary sclerosing cholangitis	
Labs	- CRP > ESR - Fecal calprotectin > lactoferrin - p-ANCA + (Myeloperoxidase)	- CRP/ESR less commonly elevated - Fecal calprotectin (if colon Dz) - ASCA +
Imaging	Toxic megacolon (≥ 6 cm) more common, diffuse colonic thickening, non-sp.	Toxic megacolon less common, String sign (distal ileum narrowing), bowel wall thickening, skip lesions
Scope Findings	- Rectal ulceration, spreads proximally - Continuous erythema, friability	- Rectum spared, perirectal fistulas - Anywhere in GIT, terminal ileum most common - Skip lesions
Path	Superficial ulcer w/ crypt abscesses (architectural distortion)	Deep ulcers with granulomas (architectural distortion)
Cancer	+ + +	+
Repeat Scope	After 8 years, then every 1-2 years	
Rx	1. 5-ASA (mesalamine) 800-1600 mg PO TID x 6 wk +/- 2. Prednisone 40-60 mg PO qd OR Methylprednisolone 40-60 mg IV BID 3. Consider biologics (hepatitis panel, Gold Quantiferon 1st) 4. Consider 6-mercaptopurine + Azathioprine to spare steroids/resistant	
	- Add 5-ASA PR qhs to q3h if rectal Dz (enema if able to hold 15-30 min, supp if not - Steroid + Cipro/Flagyl if toxic megacolon, +/- hydrocortisone enema Sx if not better in 24h - Severe if >10 BM/d, bloody, SIRS criteria	- Sx C/S & Cipro/Flagyl if perianal - TPN if unable to tolerate PO - Check iron studies, B12

Nephrology & Urology

Hyponatremia

(< 135 mEq/L)

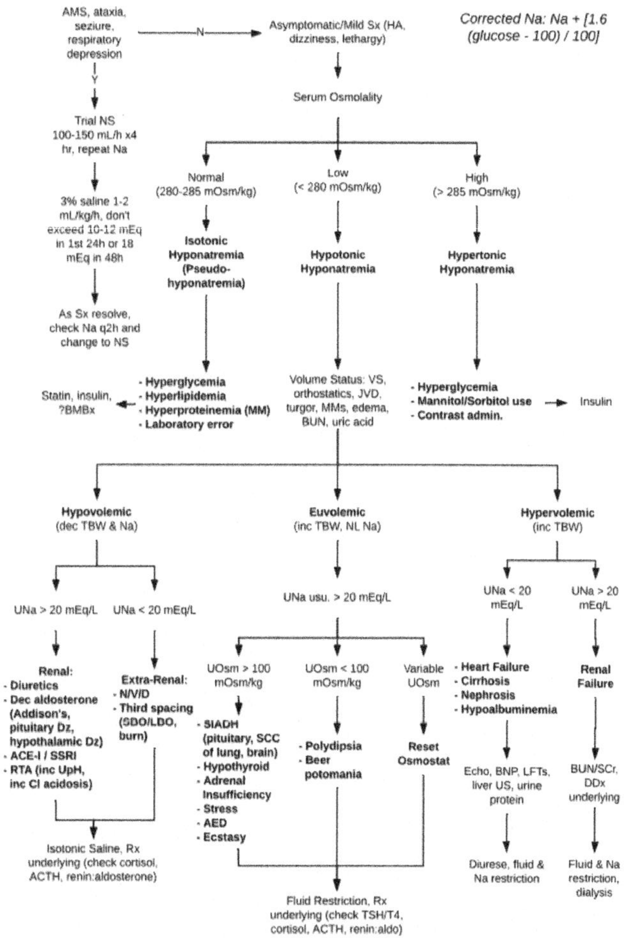

Hypernatremia

(> 145 mEq/L)

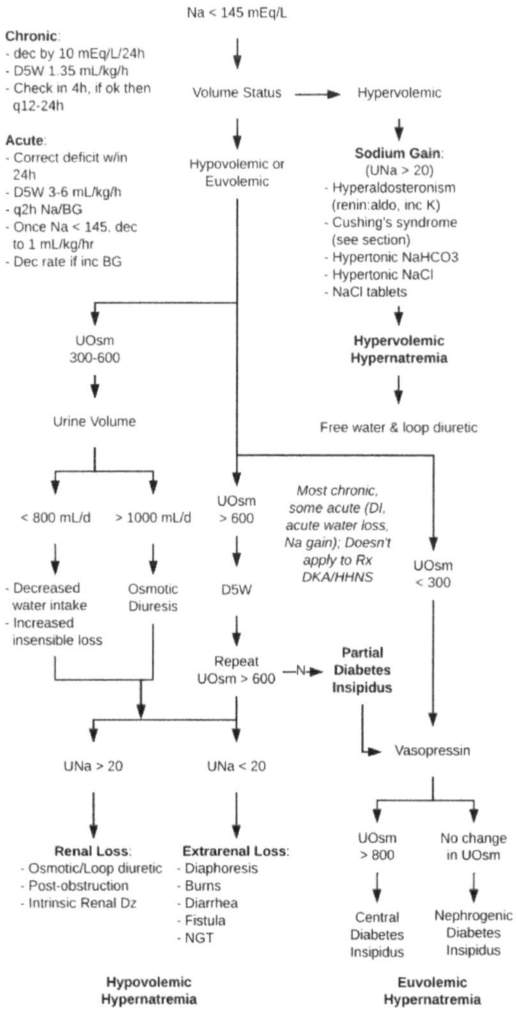

Hypokalemia

(< 3.5 mEq/L) ***Inhibitory***

Manifestations:

- Shallow respirations
- Muscular weakness /cramps & fatigue
- Lethargy
- Constipation or ileus d/t SM involvement
- EKG w/ ↓ amplitude, shallow/broad T waves, prominent U waves
- PVCs, VT/VF
- If severe (e.g., < 2.5 mEq/L)
  - Flaccid paralysis
  - Tetany
  - Hyporeflexia
  - Rhabdomyolysis

Management:

- > 2.5 mEq/L w/out EKG abnormalities
  - Tolerates PO → PO replacement, q 10 mEq → ↑ K+ 0.1 mEq/L
  - Cannot tolerate PO, then IV @ 10 mEq/hr
- < 2.5 mEq/L or severe S/S present
  - Give K+ 40 mEq/L/hr IV
  - Check BMP q3h
  - Institute continuous EKG monitoring/ telemetry
- Check Mg if refractory & correct first!

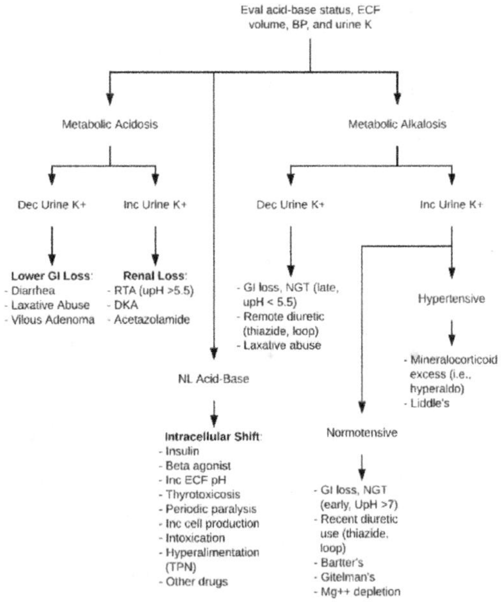

Hyperkalemia

(> 5 mEq/L) ***Excitatory***

Etiology:

- Excess intake – Hx
- Renal failure – BUN/SCr
- Drugs – Hx NSAIDs, ACE-I, ARBs
- Hypoaldosteronism (ACTH/Cortisol/renin:aldo)
- Cell death – Chemo/rad (TLS), hemolysis, rhabdomyolysis
- Acidosis (DKA, ESRD)
  - K+ moves to ECF, H+ moves to ICF
  - K+ ↑ 0.7 mEq/L w/ each ↓ 0.1 pH

Diagnostics:

- EKG not sensitive – 50% pts w/ K+ > 6.5 mEq will not have EKG changes
- However, classic tall, peaked T waves may be noted

Manifestations:

- Muscle twitches → cramps → paresthesia
- Irritability/anxiety
- Abdominal cramping
- Diarrhea

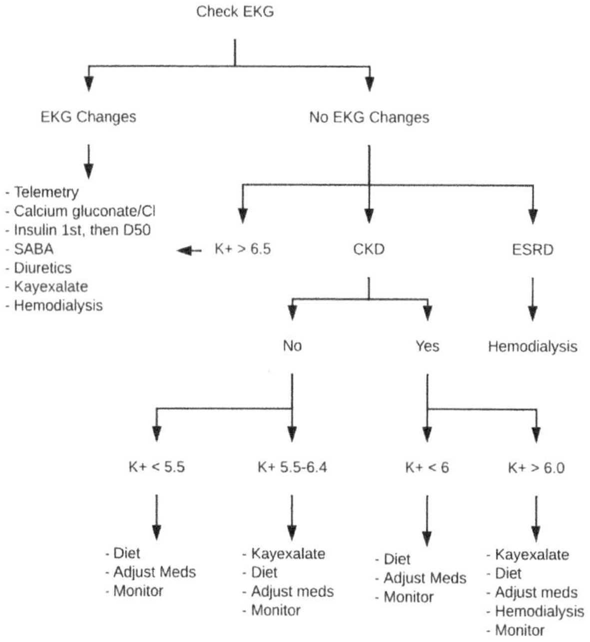

Hypocalcemia

(< 8.5 mg/dL, < 4.5 mg/dL)

Excitatory

Etiology:

- Hypoparathyroidism – PTH
- Hypomagnesemia – Mg level
- Pancreatitis – amylase/lipase
- Renal failure – BUN/SCr
- Severe trauma – Hx, MOI
- Multiple blood transfusions – Hx
- Vitamin D deficiency – Vit D level

Manifestations:

- ↑ DTRs
- Muscle/abd cramps
- Carpopedal spasm (**Trousseau's**)
- Facial spasm (**Chvostek**)
- Convulsions
- Prolonged QTI

Management:

- Check pH, look for alkalosis
- Nutrition – dairy, leafy greens, fish, nuts
- If acute, then IV
  - Calcium gluconate 1-3 g IV q6h prn
  - Calcium chloride 500-1000 mg IV q4-6h prn
- If chronic, then PO
  - Calcium carbonate 500 mg PO TID/QID
  - Vitamin D 1500-2000 units PO daily ?6000 units PO daily x 8 weeks
  - If hyperphosphatemia, then aluminum hydroxide 300-600 mg PO TID w/ meals

See Hypoparathyroidism

Hypercalcemia

(> 10.5 mg/dL, 5.5 mg/dL)

Inhibitory

Etiology:

- Hyperparathyroidism – PTH
- Hyperthyroidism – TSH/T4
- Vitamin D intoxication – Vit D level
- Prolonged immobilization – Hx, CK
- Thiazide diuretics – Hx

Manifestations:

- Fatigability
- Muscle weakness
- Depression
- Anorexia
- N/V/C
- ↓ DTRs
- AMS/lethargy
- Severe ↑ Ca can cause coma/death

Management:

- D/C Ca/Vit D supplements & thiazides
- NS infusion w/ loop diuretics
- Bisophosphonates – ↓ bone reabsorption
  - Pamidronate 60-90 mg IV x1, repeat in 7 days
  - Etidronate 20 mg/kg PO daily x30 d
- Calcium binders
- Calcitonin if impaired CV or renal Fx
- Phosphate salts as last resort
  - K-phos
  - Neutra-phos
- May need dialysis
- If > 12 mg/dL, then emergent

See Hyperparathyroidism

Hypomagnesemia

(< 1.5 mg/dL)

Excitatory

Etiology:

- UGI loss/diarrhea/ steatorrhea
- Malabsorption condition
- ↓ intake (starvation, ETOH, NGT, PPI)
- Renal Loss (diuretics, aminoglycosides, amphotericin B)
- Parathyroidectomy (Hungry bone syndrome)

Manifestations:

- GI
  - Paralytic ileus
  - N/V
  - Anorexia/ constipation
- CNS
  - Psychological depression
  - Psychosis
  - Confusion
- Neuromuscular
  - Hyperactive DTRs
  - Paresthesia
  - Muscle spasms (charley horse)

Management:

- Isolate cause
- D/C pharmacologic Contributors
- Repletion (Mg gluconate, chloride, sulfonate, oxide)

Hypermagnesemia

(> 2.6 mg/dL)

Inhibitory

Etiology:

- Antacids
- Laxatives
- Excessive Mg++ replacement
- ↓ renal function

Manifestations:

- CV when > 4 mg/dL
  - Peripheral vasodilation
  - Hypotension
  - Prolonged PRI
  - Widened QRS complex
  - Low DBP
- CNS
  - ↓ nerve impulse transmission
  - Drowsy/lethargic
- Neuromuscular
  - ↓ DTRs
  - Progressively weaker skeletal muscle contraction

Management:

- Mimics treatments for hyperkalemia
- Insulin/D50/IVF
- Discontinue supplements
- Loop diuretics
- Dialysis
- Prevention (cautious repletion)

Correct Magnesium deficiency **BEFORE** Potassium and Calcium!

Hypophosphatemia

(< 3 mg/dL)

Inhibitory

General:

- Effects d/t ↓ energy metabolism
- Clinical signs d/t hypercalcemia (b/c reciprocal relationship)

Etiology:

- Renal wasting (hyper-parathyroidism, renal failure, Fanconi's syndrome, tyrosine kinase inhibitors)
- ↓ absorption (vit D deficiency, malabsorption, alcoholism, phosphate binders (Ca carbonate), hyperalimentation
- ↑ cell uptake (Rx of DKA, carb repletion in ETOH – refeeding syndrome)

Manifestations:

- AMS/lethargy/coma
- Muscle weakness
- ↓ DTRs
- Constipation/anorexia
- N/V
- Paralytic ileus
- ↑ DVTs
- Mild Bx changes
- Polyuria/polydipsia
- Tachycardia → bradycardia
- HTN

Management:

- Dietary replacement
- PO/PT – K phos/Neutra-phos
- IV – sodium phosphate/potassium phosphate
- Caution w/ IV repletion
    - Not to exceed 7 mmol/hr
    - K/Na supplementation (monitor)

Hyperphosphatemia

(> 4.5 mg/dL)

Excitatory

General:

- Typically well-tolerated
- Effects d/t hypocalcemia (b/c reciprocal relationship)

Etiology:

- ↓ renal excretion
- Tumor lysis syndrome
- ↑ pharmacologic/ dietary intake
- Hypoparathyroidism

Manifestations:

- Bradycardia
- Hypotension
- EKG changes
    - Prolonged STI
    - Prolonged QTI

Management:

- Dietary restrictions
- Oral phosphate binders
    - Phoslo (calcium acetate)
    - Renagel (Sevelamer)
    - Alucaps (aluminum hydroxide – base for antacids)
- Must be given with food
- IVF in severe cases

Acid-Base

pH (7.4) / $PaCO_2$ (40) / HCO_3^- (24)

#1 Determine the Primary Problem

Start looking only @ pH & $PaCO_2$

ROME = Respiratory opposite, Metabolic equal.

Same direction = Metabolic

Low pH = Acidosis

High pH = Alkalosis

Vomiting (↓ Cl), Cl responsive (NaCl)

Cushing's (excess adrenocortical hormone), not responsive

Opposite direction = Respiratory

Low pH = Acidosis

High pH = Alkalosis

#2 Determine Compensation

Metabolic Acidosis = Low pH & Low $PaCO_2$

$PaCO_2 = 1.5(HCO_3^-) + 8$

Metabolic Alkalosis = High pH & High $PaCO_2$

$PaCO_2$: Baseline $PaCO_2$ ($bPaCO_2$) + 0.7 (Change HCO_3^-)

Respiratory Acidosis = Low pH & High $PaCO_2$

10:1 ratio (acute): AECOPD, narcotics

10:3.5 (chronic): Chronic COPD, chronic CO_2 retainer if HCO_3 high

E.g., 40 (24) --> 50 (25/27.5) --> 60 (26/31)

Respiratory Alkalosis = High pH & Low $PaCO_2$

10:2 (acute): Early asthma

10:5 (chronic): Pregnancy, progesterone = resp. stimulant

#3 Determine Anion Gap

(Na - Cl - CO2 = Anion Gap, NL ~12)

Metabolic Acidosis + Gap = AGMA

G - Glycols (Ethylene [stones], Propylene [Lorazepam])

O - Oxoproline (from paracetamol/acetaminophen)

L - L-lactate (sepsis, seizure, metformin)

D - D-lactate (GI)

M - Methanol (formic acid): Fumaric acid --> Proton --> Formate --> AG

A - ASA

R - Renal failure (ESRD, uremia)

K - Ketoacidosis (starvation, diabetic, alcoholic)

Metabolic Acidosis w/out Gap = NAGMA

U – Ureterostomy

S – Small bowel fistula or Rou En Y (GI Sx)

E – Extra chloride

D – Diarrhea

C – Carbonic anhydrase inhibitors

A – Addison's Dz (hyper K+)

R – RTA, esp. type 1

P - Pancreatic fistulas

#4 Determine Delta Gap

X - 12 = delta gap

24 - HCO3 = delta bicarb

Delta AG / Delta HCO3

< 1, additional NAGMA

> 2, additional metabolic alkalosis

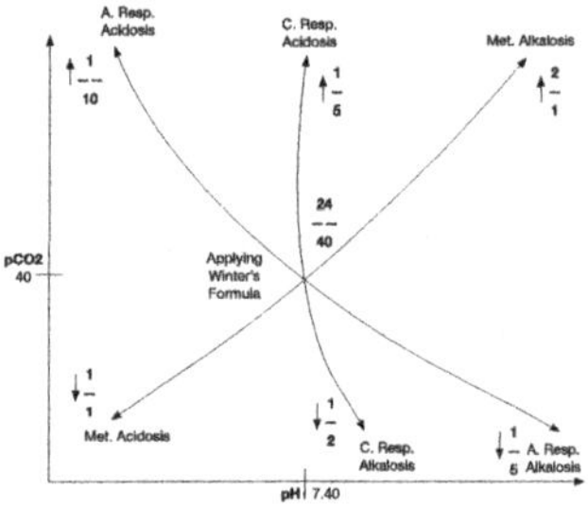

Acute/Chronic Respiratory Acidosis

- See Pulmonary section
- Lungs (asthma = ominous)
- Brainstem
- Spinal Cord
- Peripheral Nerves
- MSK/NMJ

Acute/Chronic Respiratory Alkalosis

- Early Asthma (acute)
- Progesterone = resp. stim (pregnant, OCP, cirrhosis)
- High altitude, PNA, PE
- Salicylate (resp center), Xanthines
- CNS tumor/trauma
- Anxiety/ascites

Metabolic Alkalosis

U Cl < 15

- Remote diuretics
- Volume depletion **
- Vomiting/NGT aspiration
- Exogenous alkali

U Cl > 15

- Diuretics
- Recent high BP
- Hyperaldosteronism
- Cushing's syndrome
- Licorice ingestion
- Liddle's, Gitelman's, Bartter's

Low/NL BP

- Low Mg/K
- Bartter's syndrome
- Gitelman's syndrome

Renal Tubular Acidosis (RTA)

	Proximal RTA, Type II	Distal RTA, Type IV	Classic Distal RTA, Type I
Defect	Reabsorption of HCO_3^-	H & K excretion	H excretion
Diseases	- Fanconi's - MM - Acetazolamide - Zonisamide - Topiramate - Osteomalacia	- Hypo aldosteronism - Diabetes mellitus	- Sjogren's - SLE - Stones - Obstruction - Amphotericin B
Stones	+/-	-	+
Serum K	↓	↑	↓
U pH	< 5.5 / > 5.5, Cl excreted as NH_4Cl	< 5.5	> 5.5

Bartter's	Gitelman's	Liddle's
↓ transportation defect in ascending loop of Henle	↓ transportation defect in distal tubule	↑ (aldosterone independent) transport defect in distal tubule
Low/NL BP	Low/NL BP	HTN
Hypokalemia	Hypokalemia	Hypokalemia
Urine Cl > 15	Urine Cl > 15	Urine Cl > 15
Loop diuretics	Thiazide diuretics	

Dysuria

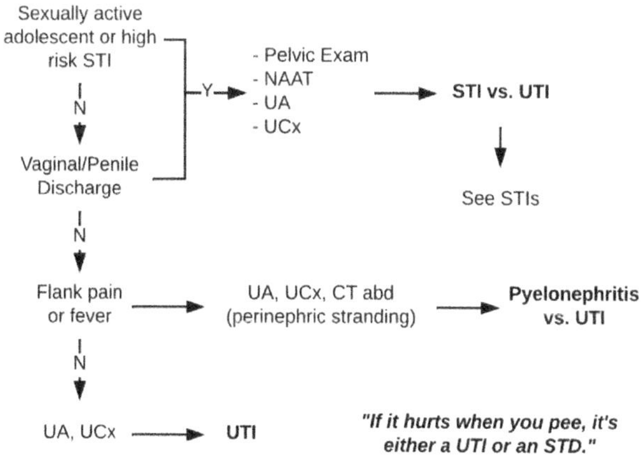

Flank Pain

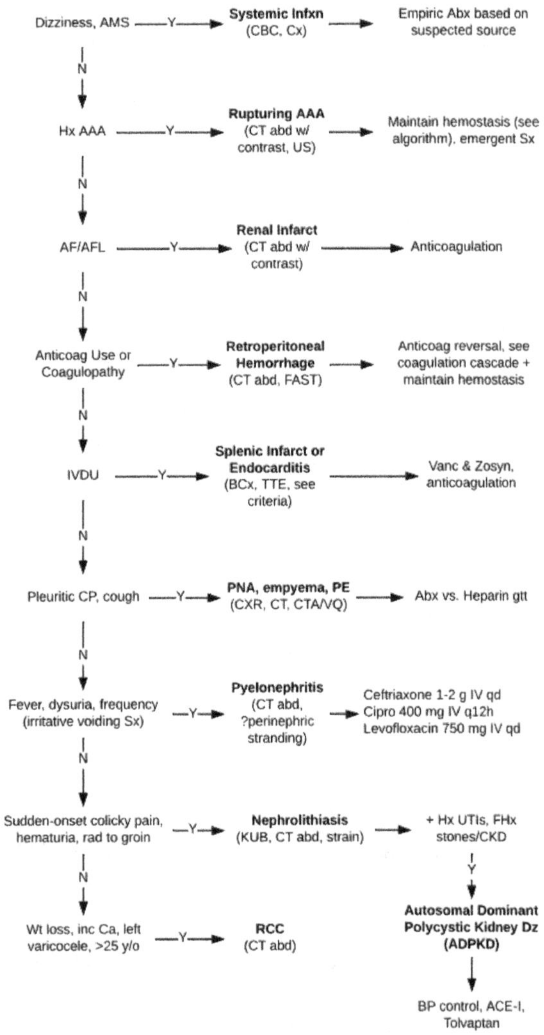
Dizziness, AMS
Y
Systemic Infxn
(CBC, Cx)
Empiric Abx based on suspected source
N
Hx AAA
Y
Rupturing AAA
(CT abd w/ contrast, US)
Maintain hemostasis (see algorithm), emergent Sx
N
AF/AFL
Y
Renal Infarct
(CT abd w/ contrast)
Anticoagulation
N
Anticoag Use or Coagulopathy
Y
Retroperitoneal Hemorrhage
(CT abd, FAST)
Anticoag reversal, see coagulation cascade + maintain hemostasis
N
IVDU
Y
Splenic Infarct or Endocarditis
(BCx, TTE, see criteria)
Vanc & Zosyn, anticoagulation
N
Pleuritic CP, cough
Y
PNA, empyema, PE
(CXR, CT, CTA/VQ)
Abx vs. Heparin gtt
N
Fever, dysuria, frequency (irritative voiding Sx)
Y
Pyelonephritis
(CT abd, ?perinephric stranding)
Ceftriaxone 1-2 g IV qd
Cipro 400 mg IV q12h
Levofloxacin 750 mg IV qd
N
Sudden-onset colicky pain, hematuria, rad to groin
Y
Nephrolithiasis
(KUB, CT abd, strain)
+ Hx UTIs, FHx stones/CKD
Y
Autosomal Dominant Polycystic Kidney Dz (ADPKD)
BP control, ACE-I, Tolvaptan
N
Wt loss, inc Ca, left varicocele, >25 y/o
Y
RCC
(CT abd)

Urinalysis

Urinary Tract Infection Evaluation

Parameter	Usual Range	Interpretation	Accuracy
Bacteria	Absent	Any amount $>10^5$ CFU/mL or 100k CFU/mL	Low sensitivity High specificity
Leukocyte Esterase	Absent	+ = pyuria, presence of WBCs in urine	High sensitivity Low specificity
WBCs	< 5	Pyuria if > 10 leukocytes/mL	High sensitivity Low specificity
Nitrite	Absent	+ = presence of bacteria	Low sensitivity High specificity
Epithelial cells	< 5	< 5 = good sample	High = contamination
pH	4.5 – 8.0	pH ↑ if urea-splitting organism	Low specificity

Pyuria DDx	Eosinophiluria DDx
- Tubular injury - Interstitial Nephritis - UTI - Pyelonephritis	- Acute interstitial nephritis (AIN) - Atheroembolism - Rapidly proliferative glomerulonephritis - Acute prostatitis

Cast & UA Finding DDx

Type of Cast/UA Finding	Correlation
Hyaline casts	Pre-renal azotemia (dehydration, diuretic) ** Nephrotic syndrome
RBC casts	Nephritis, glomerular Dz
NL Erythrocytes	Lower urinary tract lesion
Dysmorphic erythrocytes	Upper urinary tract lesion
Fatty casts/Oval fat bodies	Nephrotic
Muddy/dirty brown or pigmented	Acute tubular necrosis (ATN)
Waxy, granular, cellular casts	Advanced chronic renal Dz
Leukocyte casts + eosinophils	Acute interstitial nephritis (AIN)
Leukocytes, leukocyte casts + bacteriuria	Urinary tract infection (UTI)
Leukocytes, leukocyte casts – bacteriuria	Renal interstitial disease

UA w/ WBCs, no casts, +polyuria/nocturia, - dysuria/flank pain, Rx Abx... repeat UA +WBCs, renal US w/ 1 kidney smaller than other, IVP w/ multiple strictures → check urine for AFB or PPD to R/O renal TB

Proteinuria

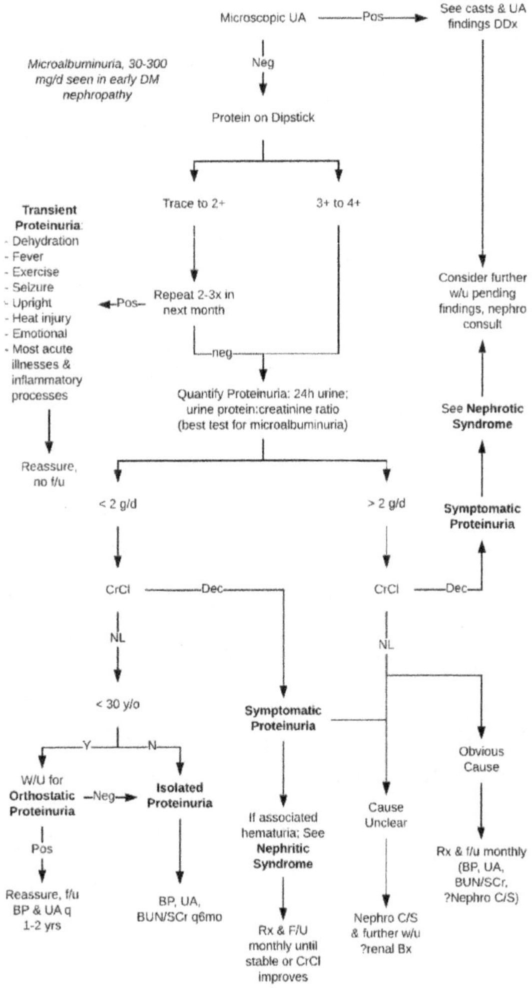

Hematuria

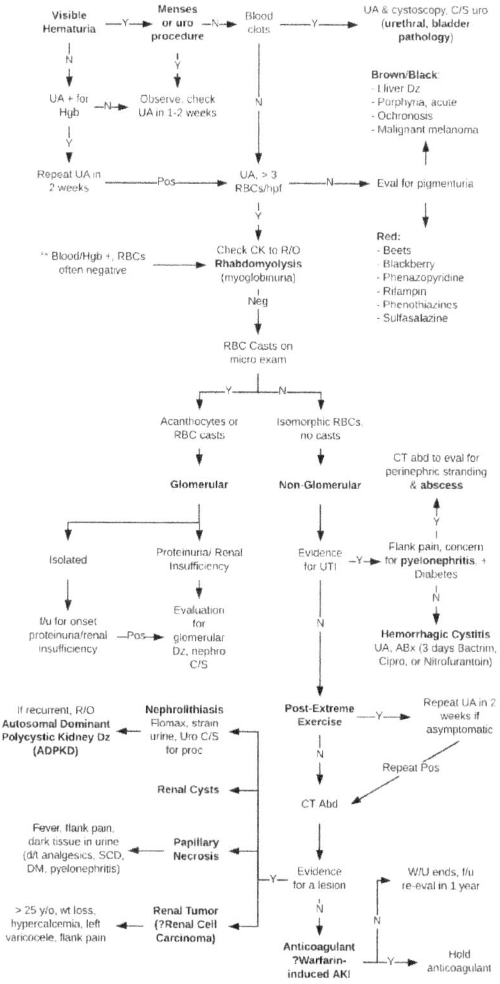

Visible Hematuria
Menses or uro procedure
Blood clots
UA & cystoscopy, C/S uro (urethral, bladder pathology)
UA + for Hgb
Observe, check UA in 1-2 weeks
Brown/Black:
- Liver Dz
- Porphyria, acute
- Ochronosis
- Malignant melanoma
Repeat UA in 2 weeks
Pos
UA, > 3 RBCs/hpf
Eval for pigmenturia
** Blood/Hgb +, RBCs often negative
Check CK to R/O Rhabdomyolysis (myoglobinuria)
Neg
Red:
- Beets
- Blackberry
- Phenazopyridine
- Rifampin
- Phenothiazines
- Sulfasalazine
RBC Casts on micro exam
Acanthocytes or RBC casts
Isomorphic RBCs, no casts
Glomerular
Non-Glomerular
CT abd to eval for perinephric stranding & abscess
Isolated
Proteinuria/ Renal Insufficiency
Evidence for UTI
Flank pain, concern for pyelonephritis, + Diabetes
f/u for onset proteinuria/renal insufficiency
Evaluation for glomerular Dz, nephro C/S
Hemorrhagic Cystitis
UA, ABx (3 days Bactrim, Cipro, or Nitrofurantoin)
If recurrent, R/O Autosomal Dominant Polycystic Kidney Dz (ADPKD)
Nephrolithiasis
Flomax, strain urine, Uro C/S for proc
Post-Extreme Exercise
Repeat UA in 2 weeks if asymptomatic
Repeat Pos
Renal Cysts
CT Abd
Fever, flank pain, dark tissue in urine (d/t analgesics, SCD, DM, pyelonephritis)
Papillary Necrosis
Evidence for a lesion
W/U ends, f/u re-eval in 1 year
> 25 y/o, wt loss, hypercalcemia, left varicocele, flank pain
Renal Tumor (?Renal Cell Carcinoma)
Anticoagulant ?Warfarin-induced AKI
Hold anticoagulant

Acute Kidney Injury (AKI)

Rapid impairment in kidney function → sudden ↓ in GFR → retention of metabolic waste products and dysregulation of fluid, electrolyte, and acid-base homeostasis

Stage	SCr Criteria	UOP Criteria
I	1.5 x or > 0.3 mg/dL	UO < 0.5 mL/kg/h x 6 h
II	2 x	UO < 0.5 mL/kg/h x 12 h
III	3 x or RRT	UO < 0.3 mL/kg/h x 24 h or anuria x 12 h

Pre-Renal AKI

Hypoperfusion of the kidneys (60-70% cases), if not reversed will progress to ATN

Etiology:
- Hypovolemia: hemorrhage, diuresis, N/V/D. NG suction, DKA, DI, poor PO intake, pancreatitis (shift)
- Impaired Cardiac Function: HF, dysrhythmia, cardiogenic shock, tamponade
- Vasodilation (↓ SVR): sepsis, anaphylaxis, neurogenic shock, antihypertensives
- Afferent Arteriolar Vasoconstriction: NSAIDs, contrast, hypercalcemia, hepatorenal syndrome
- Efferent Arteriolar Vasodilation: ACE-I, ARB

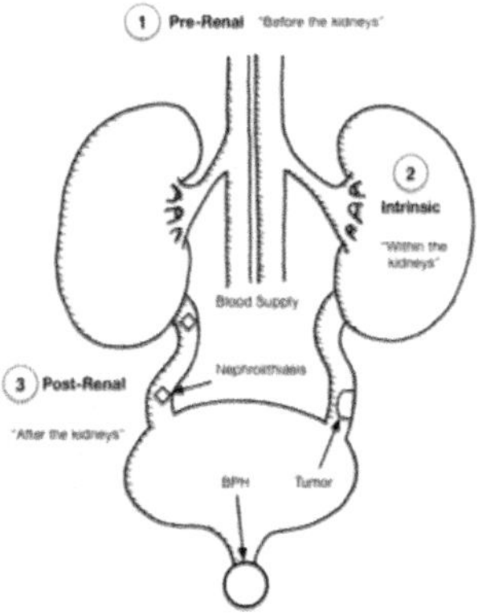

Laboratory/Diagnostic:
- Urine osmolality (UOsm) > 500, concentration of urine
- Urine sodium (UNa) < 20, still able to reabsorb Na
- BUN:SCr > 20:1, still able to reabsorb urea
- FeNa < 1.0%, FeUr < 35%
- US: NL sized kidneys

Intrinsic AKI

1. Acute Tubular Necrosis (ATN)
2. Acute Interstitial Neprhitis (AIN)
3. Acute Vascular Disease
4. Glomerular Disease

- Urine osmolality < 350, inability to concentrate urine
- Urine sodium > 40, inability to reabsorb sodium
- BUN:SCr < 20:1, inability to reabsorb urea
- FeNa > 1.0%, FeUr > 35%
- US: NL sized kidneys

ATN	AIN	GN, Vasculitis, MM	Rhabdomyolysis
- Renal tubular cells/casts - Epithelial casts - Pigmented casts (muddy brown, coarse)	- Eosinophils - WBC casts - WBCs	- Hematuria - RBC casts - Dysmorphic RBCs - Protein > 3.5 g	- +Blood - Port wine color - CK 10x NL

Acute Tubular Necrosis (ATN)

Caused by prolonged ischemia r/t poor perfusion or nephrotoxin (drug or pigment)

Nephrotoxins: ACE-I, ARBs, contrast, Abx/Antifungals (aminoglycosides, amphotericin B, beta-lactams, quinolones, sulfonamides), diuretics, lithium, methotrexate, NSAIDs, statins, chemo, rhabdomyolysis, IV hemolysis

History supports prolonged ischemia or pigment

UA: renal tubular cells/casts, epithelial casts, pigmented casts (muddy brown, coarse)

Rhabdomyolysis: +blood, port wine color, CK 10x NL, microscopy

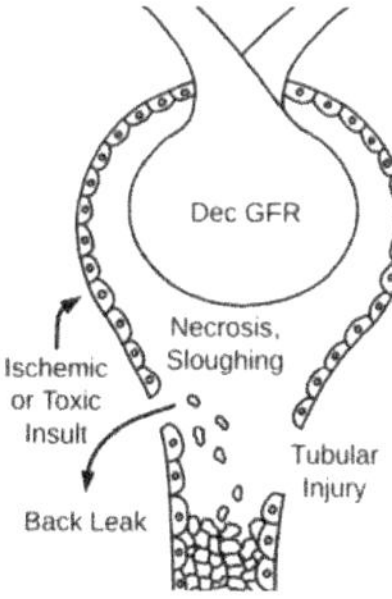

Acute Interstitial Nephritis (AIN)

Caused by allergic reaction (rash, fever, arthralgia), pyelonephritis, sarcoidosis

Consider recent med changes

UA: eosinophils, WBC casts, WBCs

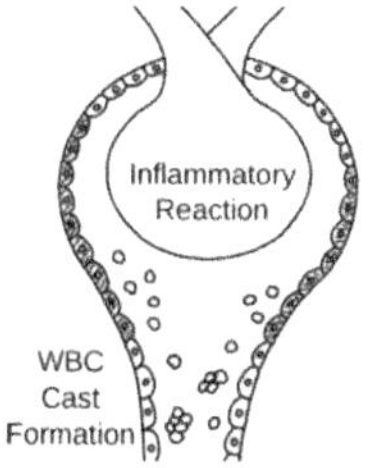

Acute Vascular Disease

- Systemic sclerosis
- Thrombotic thrombocytopenia purpura (TTP)
- Hemolytic uremic syndrome (HUS)
- Malignant HTN
- Emboli (cholesterol)
- Renal artery thrombosis/embolus
- Abdominal compartment syndrome

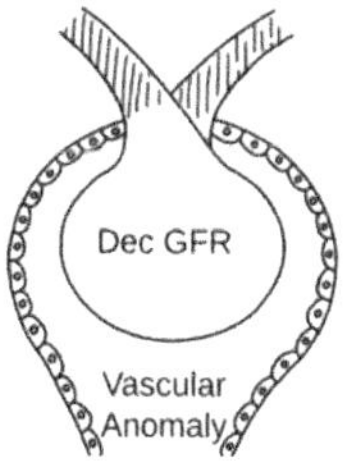

Glomerular Disease

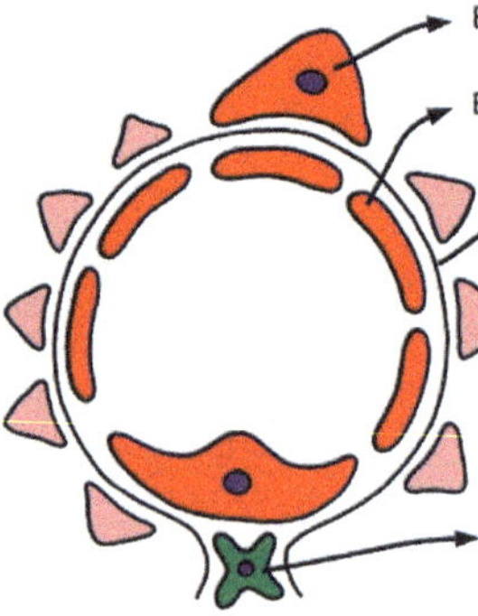

1. Know the 2 major presentations (nephrotic, nephritic)

2. Know histopathological patterns

3. Know diseases associated with histopathological patterns

Nephrotic vs. Nephritic Syndrome

Characteristic	**Nephrotic Syndrome**	**Nephritic Syndrome**
Onset	Insidious	Abrupt
Primary UA Presentation	Primarily proteinuria, >3g/d	Primarily hematuria
	+/- Hematuria	Proteinuria < 3g/d
Creatinine	Likely NL	Elevated
Casts	Fatty casts, fat oval bodies	RBC casts, cola/smoky urine
Primary Signs/Symptoms	Edema (general/periorbital), HTN	HTN

Nephrotic Syndrome

Histopathologic Presentations & Etiology

	Minimal Change	**Focal Segmental**	**Membranous**	**Membrano-proliferative (MPGN)**
Etio	- Hodgkin's - Leukemia - NSAIDs - Lithium	- African A. - HIV - Heroin - SCD - Obesity	- Hep B, C - Syphilis - Tumors - Malaria - NSAIDs - SLE - ACE-I, Gold, PCN'ine	- Hep B, C - SLE - Cryoglobulinemia (hep C +, palpable purpura, MM)
Tests	Li level, WBCs	Rapid HIV, smear	Hepatitis panel, RPR, FTA-Abs, anti-dsDNA	Hepatitis panel, SPEP, anti-dsDNA
Bx/LM	Normal	Sclerosis of part of glomerulus in few glomeruli	Thickened capillary loops	Tramtrack (double contour to many basement membranes)
IM	Normal	IgM + C3	Granular, IgG + C3	Mesangial deposit
EM	Effacement of epithelial foot processes	Effacement of epithelial foot processes	Sub-epithelial deposits, basement membrane	Ribbon/sausaging of membrane in type II, subendothelial deposits
Comp-lement	Normal	Normal	Normal	Low
Rx	Steroids, CYP	Steroids, CYP	Steroids, CYP	Steroids, CYP, +/- ASA
Diffuse Deposition: Amyloid (RA, Crohn's, MM)				

Complications

Proteinuria > 3 g/d →	Hypoalbuminemia	→ Edema
	Hypogammaglobulinemia	→ Infections
	Loss of antithrombin III, antiplasmin	→ Thrombosis & PE
	Loss of transferrin	→ IDA
	Loss of Vit D protein	→ Osteomalacia
Lipiduria →	Fat bodies, fatty casts, HLD	

Management:

- ACE-I, reduces proteinuria and HLD
- Low sodium diet
- Loop diuretics
- HMG-CoA reductase inhibitors (-statin)

Nephritic Syndrome

Histopathologic Presentations & Etiology

	Post-Strep. GN (PSGN)	IgA Nephropathy	Henoch-Schonlein Purpura (HSP)	Rapidly Proliferative GN (RPGN)
Etiology	Strep infxn 1-3 wk ago or skin infxn 3-6 wk ago	Most common post-exercise, URI < 1 wk ago (poss. Strep)	Idiopathic abd pain, palpable purpura	Goodpasture (young, female, smoker, gas station)
Tests	Clinical	Clinical	Clinical, Bx	Anti-GBM, ANCA
Bx/LM	Hypercellularity	Mesangial proliferation	Mesangial proliferation	Crescents (extracapillary) formation
IM	Lumpy bumpy (granular), IgG, IgM, C3	IgA, IgG, C3 deposit in mesangium	IgA, IgG, C3	Linear IgG
EM	Sub-epithelial deposits			Epithelial cell
Complement	Low C3, CH50, NL C4	Normal	Normal	Normal
Rx	Supportive Abx	1st ACE-I, then steroids	Supportive	Immuno-suppressants, plasmapheresis

↓ Complement (mainly Nephritic)	Complement NOT ↓

- Post-streptococcal GN
- MPGN
  o SLE (C3 > C4)
  o Cryoglobulinemia (C4 > C3)
- Subacute bacterial endocarditis (SBE)
- Atheroembolism
	- IgA nephropathy
	- Minimal change
	- Focal segmental
	- Membranous nephropathy
	- Goodpasture/Wagener's Dz (no immune deposits on renal biopsy)
	- Henoch-Schonlein nephropathy

AKI Algorithm

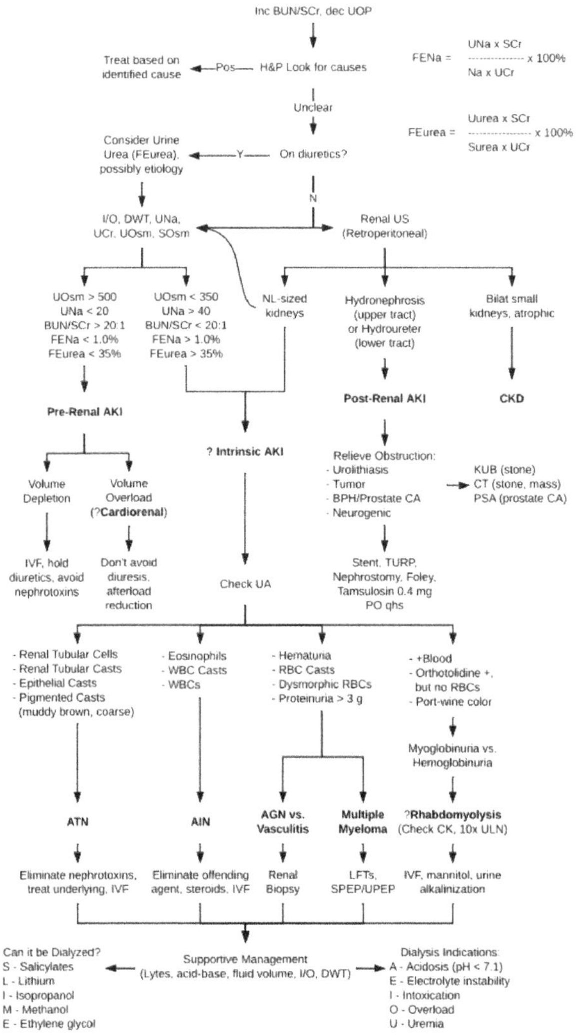

Hepatorenal Syndrome (HRS)

Presentation: Pt with Hx cirrhosis presents with elevated BUN/SCr with SBP > 140, low urine Na (suggestive), and "muddy brown casts" (hyaline casts stained by bilirubin).

Types:

- Type 1: AKI within 2 weeks
- Type 2: Subacute/insidious CKD with other causes excluded

Pathophysiology:

- "Stiff" liver —> NO release —> Splanchnic vasodilation —> poor circulatory volume —> RAAS activation
- Hepatorenal reflux hypothesis: ↑ portal pressure & sympathetic signal —> RAAS activation

Management:

- Colloid > crystalloid if volume down, albumin may bind vasodilatory factors released by cirrhotic liver
- Furosemide +/- spironolactone if volume up (CA if hyperkalemic) vs. large volume paracentesis (LVP)
- Classic Triad: Midodrine, Octreotide, Albumin – alternatively consider norepinephrine with MAP goal 85 mmHg (causes splanchnic vasoconstriction, reset's signal —> ↓ RAAS-mediated constriction of renal blood flow)

Cardiorenal Syndrome (CRS)

Presentation: Pt with Hx heart disease (arrhythmia, coronary disease, heart failure) presents with acute decompensation of heart disease and has an elevated BUN/SCr.

Types:

- Type 1: Acute HF —> AKI
- Type 2: Chronic HF —> CKD
- Type 3: Abrupt worsening of kidney Fx d/t acute cardiac dysfunction
- Type 4: Primary CKD —> cardiac dysfunction (coronary Dz, HF, arrhythmia)
- Type 5: A/C systemic Dz —> both cardiac & renal dysfunction

Dx: ↑ BUN/SCr + Cardiac precipitating factor (ADHF, coronary Dz, arrhythmia)

Rx: ↑ BUN/SCr should not deter diuresis/decongestion; aim to improve cardiac function

AKI and CKD Management

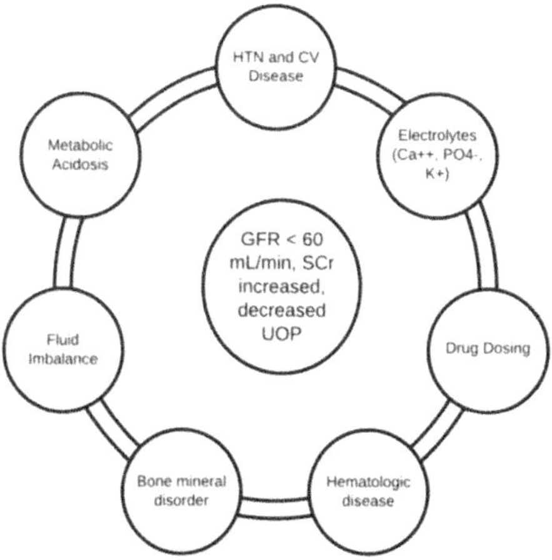

- Target underlying cause
- Fluid balance
  - DWT, I/O, IVF, BP (MAP > 65)
  - Monitor for congestion/FVO
  - 1 kg = 1 L fluid; 1 lb = 500 mL fluid
  - Diuretics, albumin
- Anemia
  - PRBCs, EPO, ferrous sulfate, iron sucrose/dextran
- Hypocalcemia
  - Ca++ carbonate (Os-Cal), Ca++ acetate (PhosLo), sevelamer HCl (Renagel)
- Hyperkalemia
  - Na polystyrene sulfonate (Kayexalate) + sorbitol
  - D50/insulin, albuterol
- Severe acidosis
  - Na+ HCO3-
- Hyperphosphatemia
  - Phosphate binding agents (calcium/lanthanum carbonate) w/ each meal
- Nephrotoxins
  - ACE-I, ARB, NSAID, RI, aminoglycoside, digoxin, phenytoin, contrast (IVF + N-acetylcysteine)
- Osteodystrophy
  - Vitamin D
- Dialysis
  - Consider when nephron Fx < 20%
  - A – Acidosis (pH < 7.1)
  - E – Electrolyte instability
  - I – Intoxication
  - O – Overload
  - U – Uremia (BUN > 100)
- Dialyzable? (**S**alicylates, **L**ithium, **I**sopropanol, **M**ethanol, **E**thylene glycol)

Genitourinary & Women's Health

Vaginal Bleeding

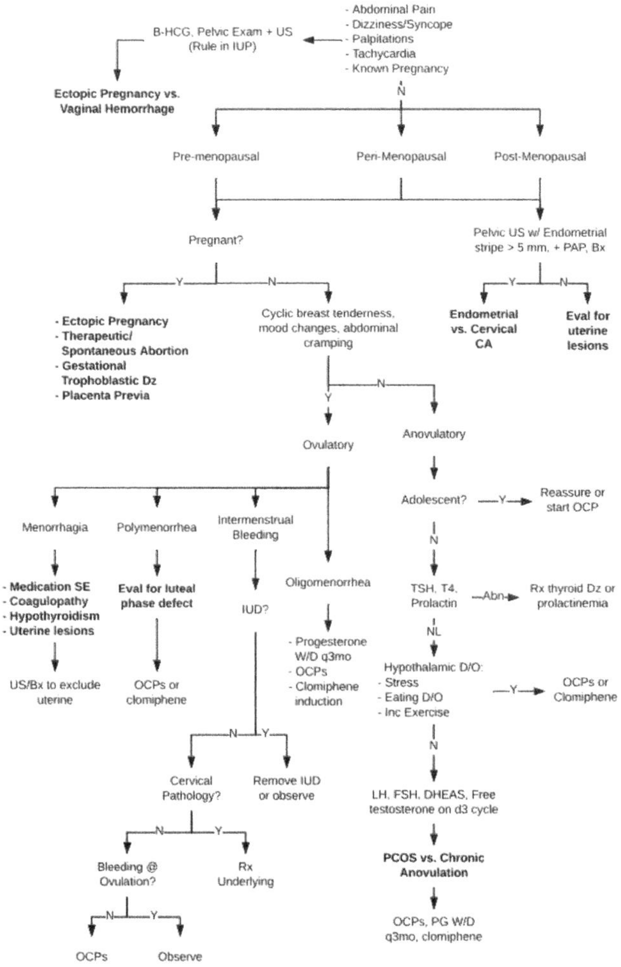

Vaginal Irritation

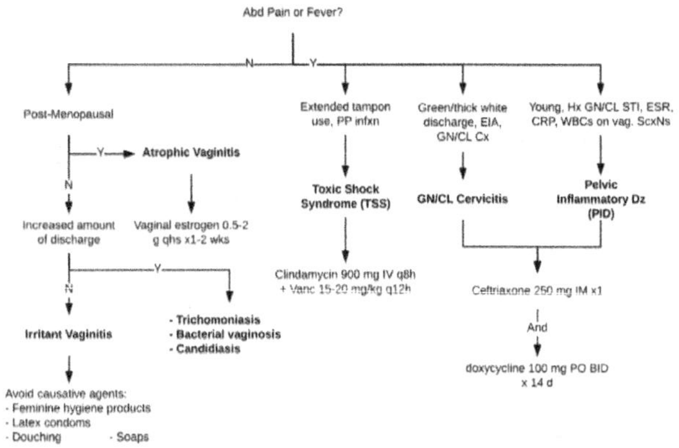

Abnormal Uterine Bleeding

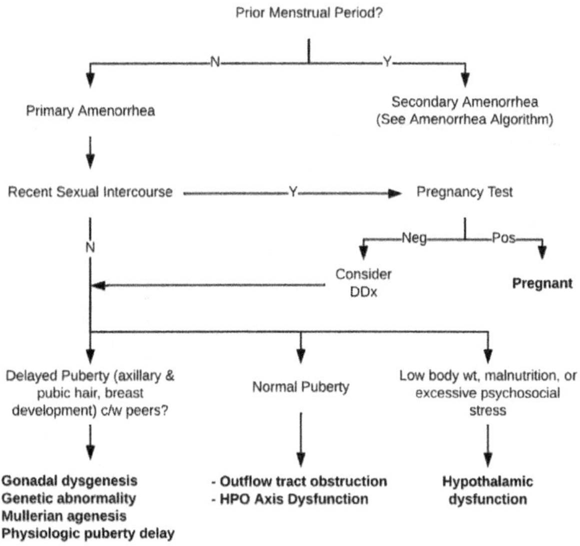

Amenorrhea

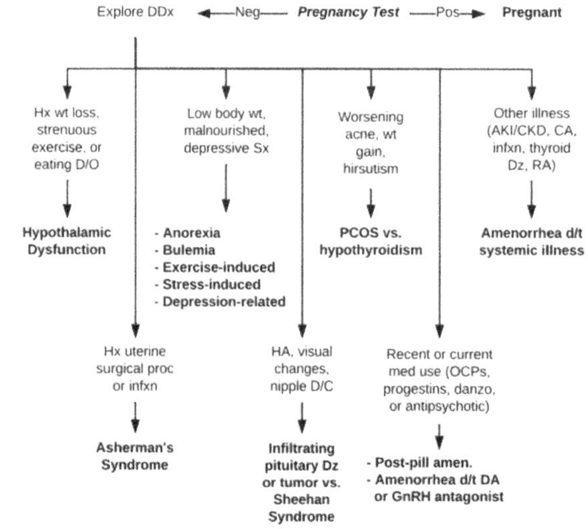

Pelvic Pain

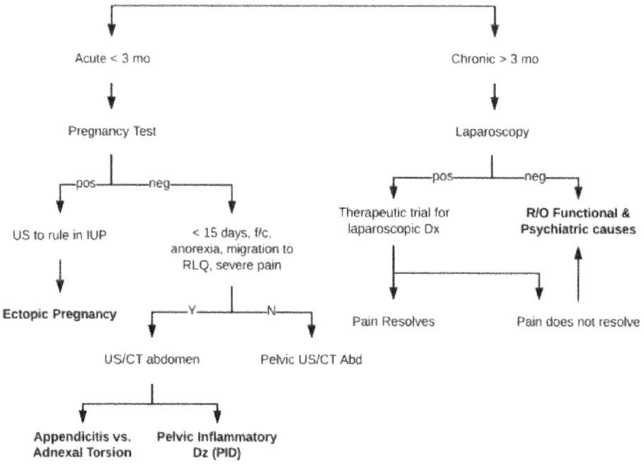

Breast Problems

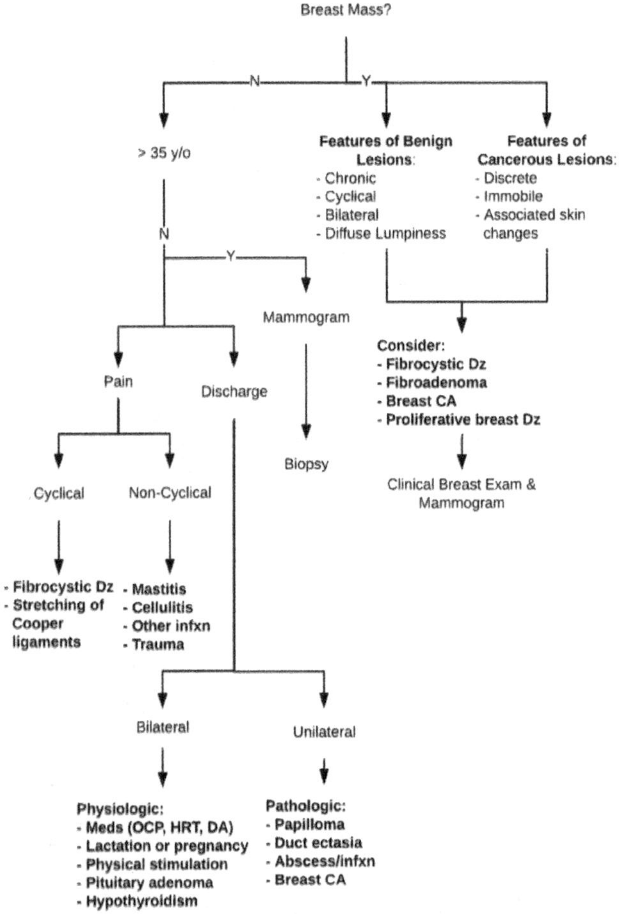

Scrotal Pain

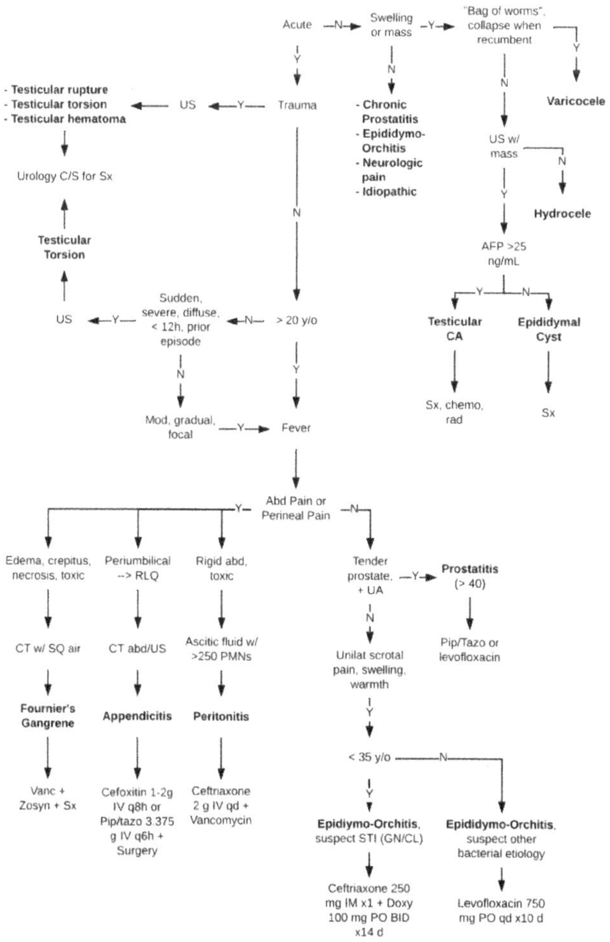

Erectile Dysfunction

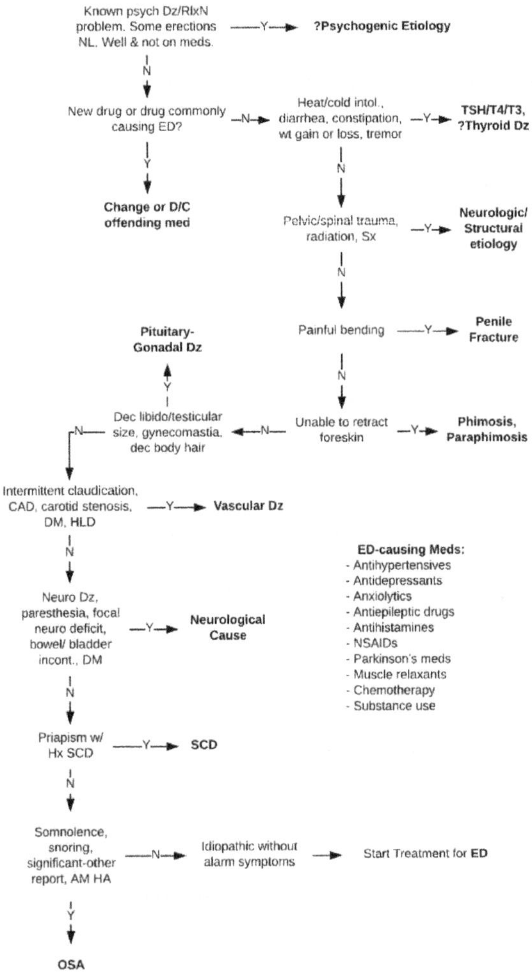

Sexually Transmitted Infections (STIs)

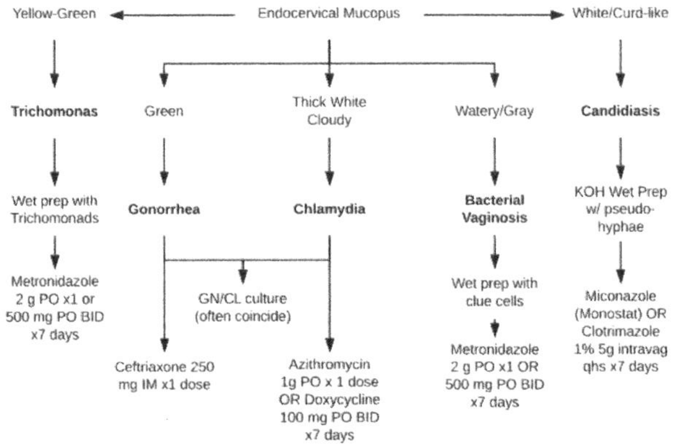

Which Ones to Report? **GCS** (Gonorrhea, Chlamydia, Syphilis)

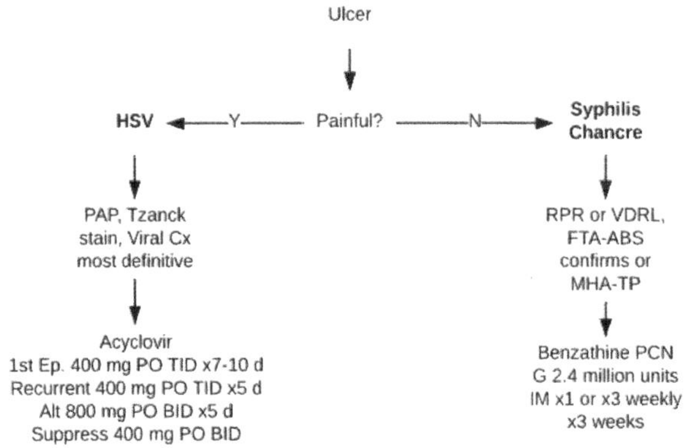

Pelvic Inflammatory Disease (PID)

Acute and subclinical infxn of upper GU tract in females. Results in endometriosis, salpingitis, oopheritis, peritonitis, perihepatitis (Fitz-Hugh Curtis syndrome), +/- tubo-ovarian abscess.

Presentation: A sexually active female (+/- partner with STI, Hx PID/STI, lack of barrier use, s/p cervical instrumentation) presents with acute BL lower abd/pelvic pain & tenderness for < 2 weeks +/- fever +/- abn uterine bleeding.

OE: Lower abd tenderness, cervical motion tenderness (Chandelier sign) and adnexal tenderness, fever/rebound/↓ BS (severe)

Workup:

- Leukocytosis, minority
- ↑ ESR/CRP (poor Se/Sp)
- Pregnancy test
- Microscopy of vaginal discharge
- NAATs for CL/GN/M. genitalium (where available)
- HIV screening, RPR, VDRL

Diagnosis:

- Presumptive based on presentation (65-90% Se), don't delay Abx!
- Additional findings supportive of PID (↑ Sp, ↓ Se)
    - Temp > 101 F
    - Abnormal cervical or vaginal mucopurulent discharge
    - More leukocytes (> 15) than epithelial cells in vaginal secretions
    - ESR > 40 or CRP > 60 (Sp 61%)
    - TVUS/CT/MRI – thickened, fluid-filled tubules/oviducts +/- free pelvic fluid, or tubo-ovarian complex OR doppler with tubal hyperemia (absence of findings does not R/O)
    - Lap with tubal erythema, edema, adhesions

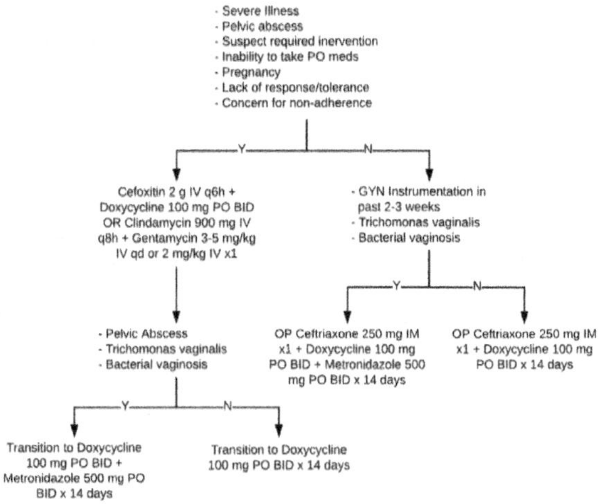

Dermatology

Common Dermatologic Lesions

Primary Lesions

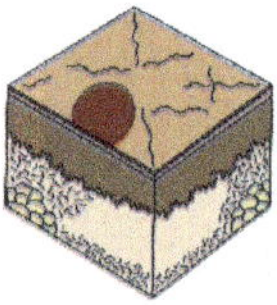

Macule: Small flat lesion < 1 cm (Freckle)

Patch: Large flat lesion > 1 cm (Birth mark)

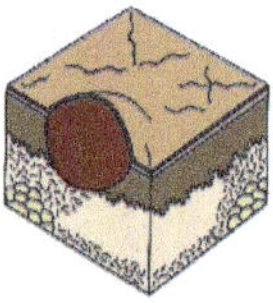

Papule: Small raised lesion < 1 cm

E.g., Allergic eczema

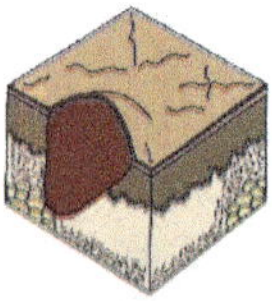

Nodule: Raised, firm, moveable < 2 cm

E.g., Mole

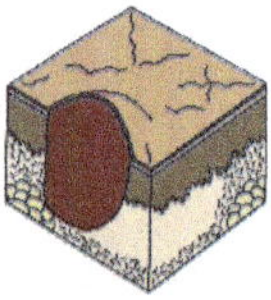

Mass: Large nodule, firm/soft, > 2 cm

E.g., squamous cell carcinoma

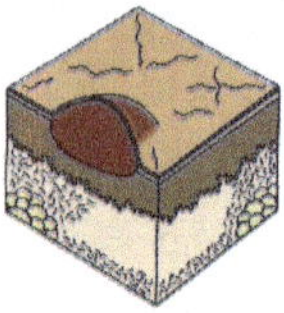

Plaque: Solid, raised, flat top, indistinct borders, > 0.5 cm

E.g., Thrush

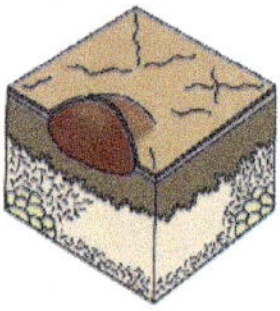

Wheal: Palpable, circumscribed edema

E.g., PPD test

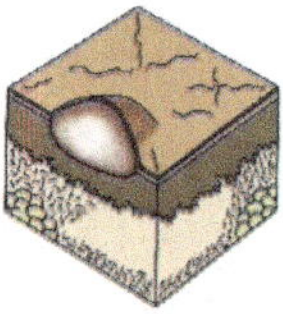

Vesicle: Raised lesion with clear fluid < 1 cm

E.g., HSV infxn

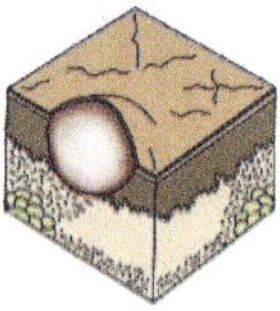

Bulla: Large fluid-filled lesion > 1 cm

E.g., Burn

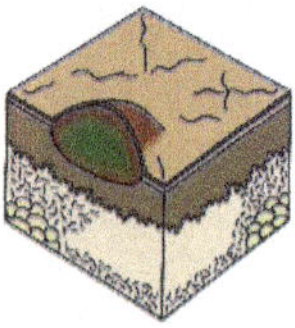

Pustule: Vesicle filled with pus

E.g., Acne

Secondary Skin Lesions

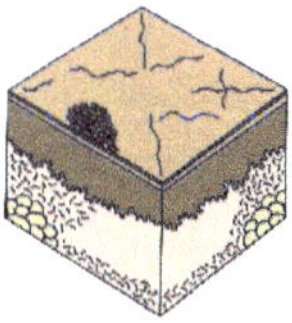

Scale: Visible shedding fragments of stratum corneum

E.g., Psoriasis

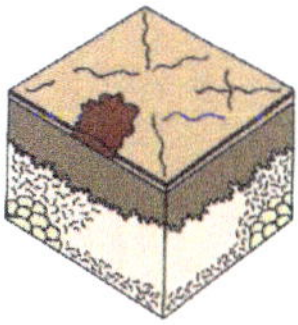

Crust: Dried exudate on skin

E.g., Impetigo

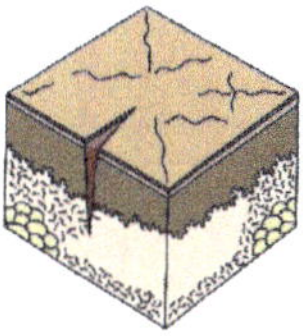

Fissure: sharply defined, linear/wedge-shaped tears in epidermis with abrupt walls

E.g., Athlete's foot

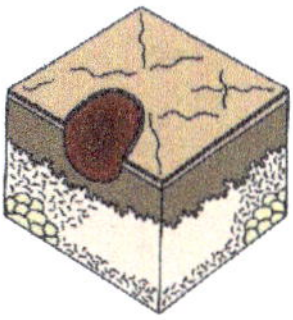

Ulcer: localized irregular areas of destruction where dermis and epidermis is lost

E.g., Decubitus

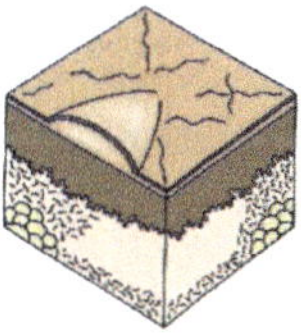

Scar: Excess collagen production after injury

E.g., surgical healing

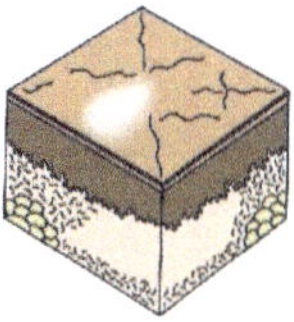

Atrophy: Loss of some portion of the skin (loss of functional units)

E.g., Paralysis

Erythematous Lesion

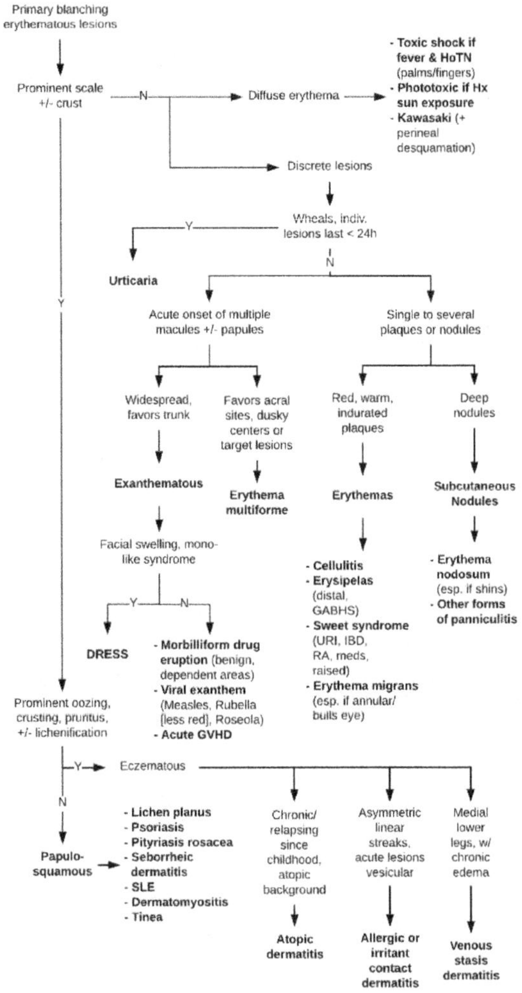

Palpable Petechiae/Purpura

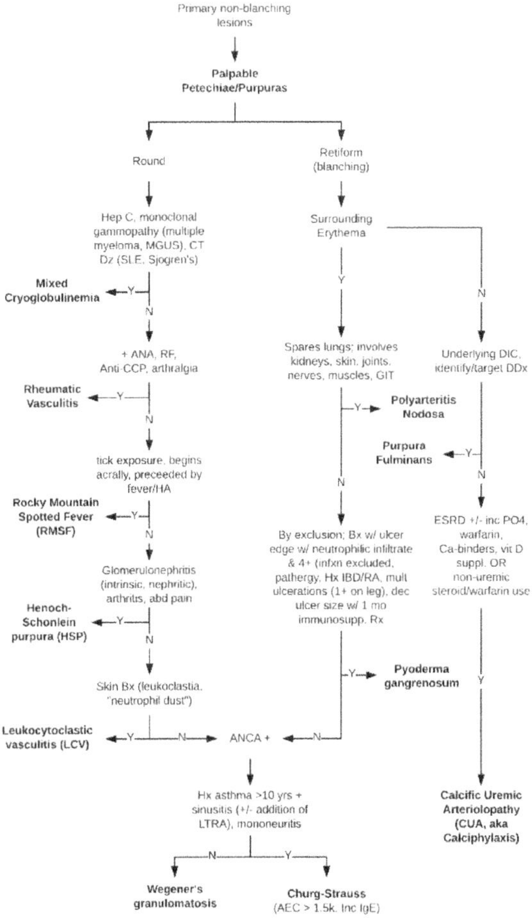

Non-Palpable Petechiae/Purpura

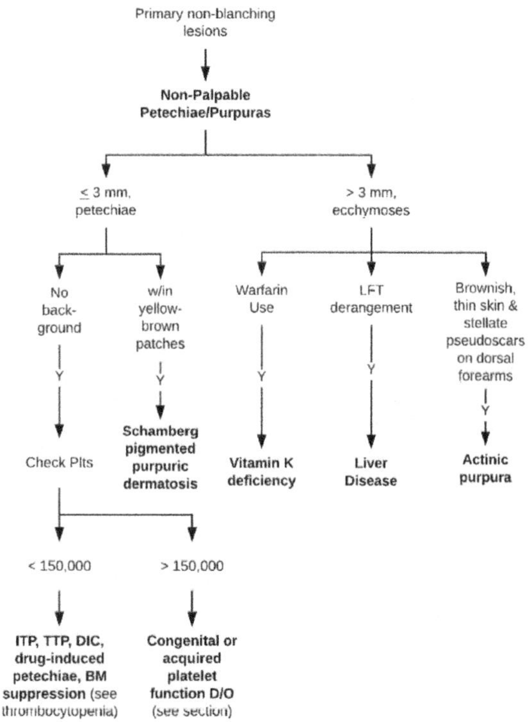

Vesicles and Pustules

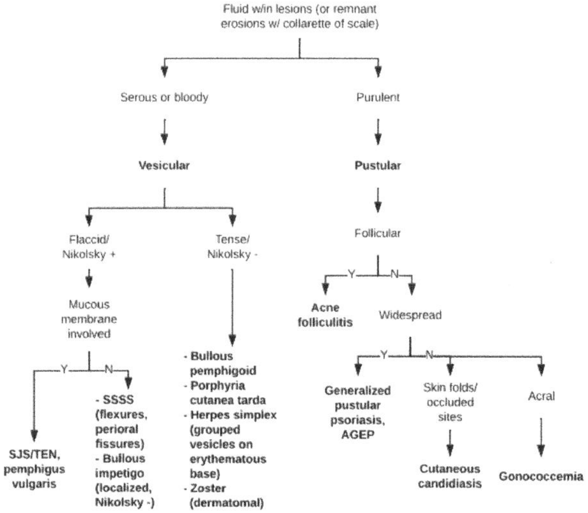

Photodistributed Macules/Patches

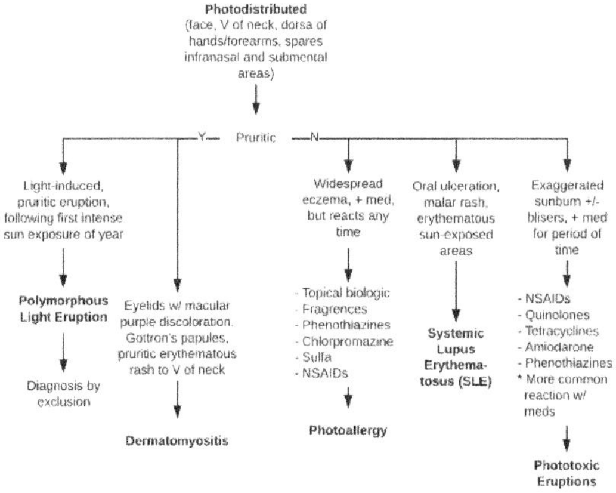

Hypopigmented Macules/Patches

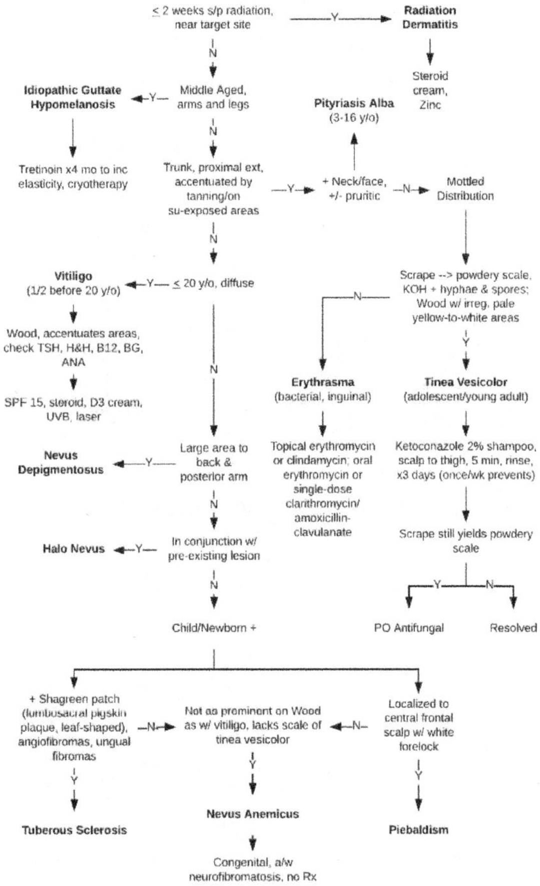

Cystic Lesion

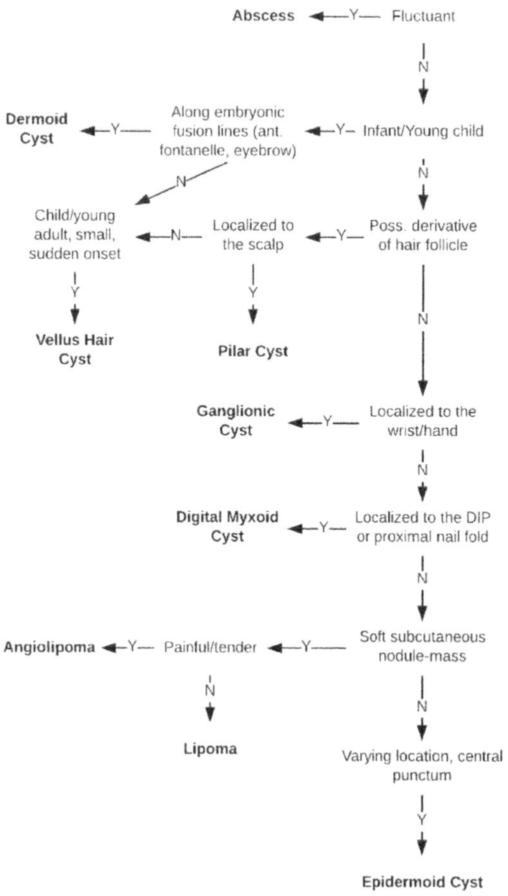

Pruritus

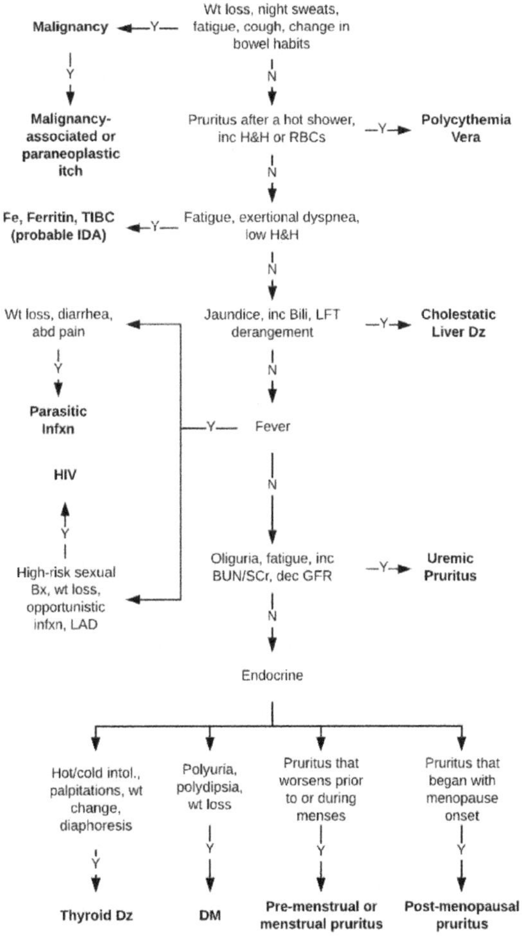
Wt loss, night sweats, fatigue, cough, change in bowel habits
Malignancy
Y
Malignancy-associated or paraneoplastic itch
N
Pruritus after a hot shower, inc H&H or RBCs
Polycythemia Vera
Fatigue, exertional dyspnea, low H&H
Fe, Ferritin, TIBC (probable IDA)
Jaundice, inc Bili, LFT derangement
Cholestatic Liver Dz
Wt loss, diarrhea, abd pain
Parasitic Infxn
Fever
HIV
High-risk sexual Bx, wt loss, opportunistic infxn, LAD
Oliguria, fatigue, inc BUN/SCr, dec GFR
Uremic Pruritus
Endocrine
Hot/cold intol., palpitations, wt change, diaphoresis
Polyuria, polydipsia, wt loss
Pruritus that worsens prior to or during menses
Pruritus that began with menopause onset
Thyroid Dz
DM
Pre-menstrual or menstrual pruritus
Post-menopausal pruritus

Cellulitis

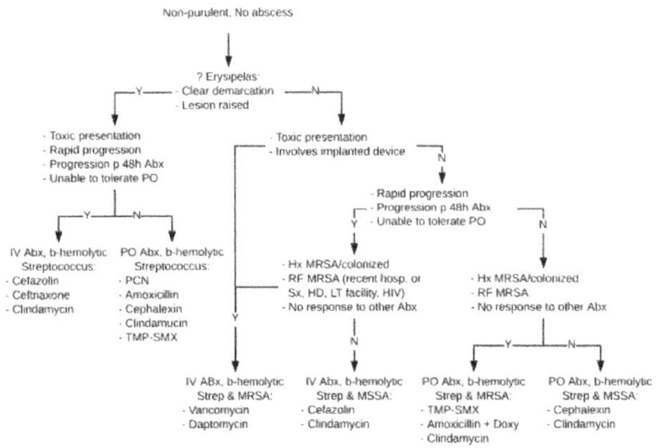

IV Cefazolin → PO Keflex **OR** IV Ampicillin/Sulbactam → PO Amoxicillin/Clavulanate

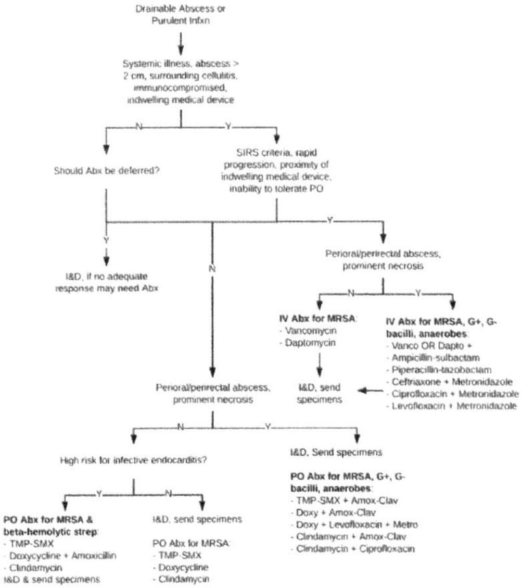

Hematology/Oncology

Anemia

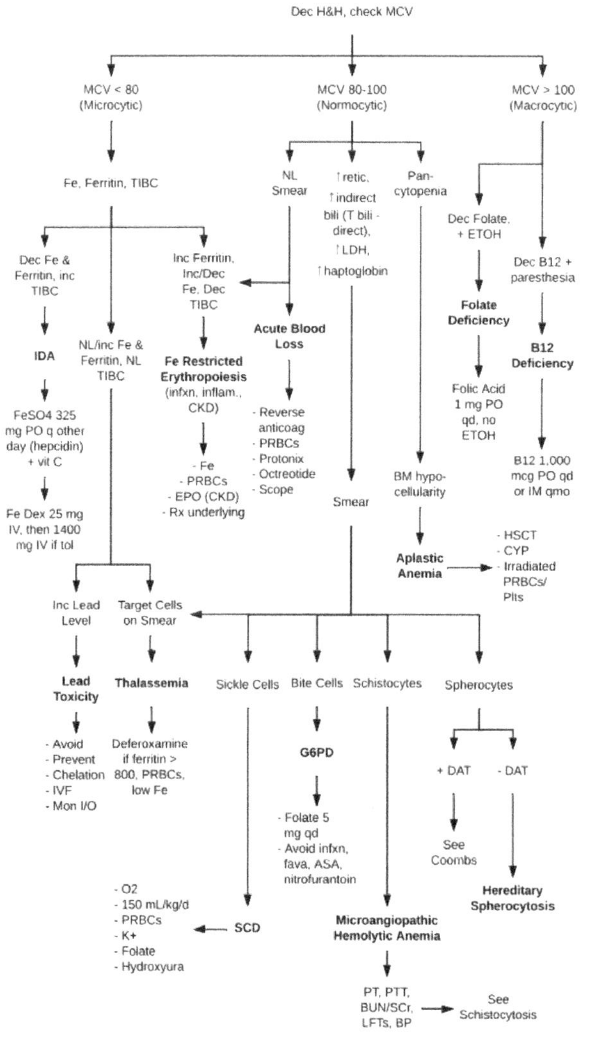
Dec H&H, check MCV
MCV < 80 (Microcytic)
MCV 80-100 (Normocytic)
MCV > 100 (Macrocytic)
Fe, Ferritin, TIBC
Dec Fe & Ferritin, inc TIBC
IDA
FeSO4 325 mg PO q other day (hepcidin) + vit C
Fe Dex 25 mg IV, then 1400 mg IV if tol
NL/inc Fe & Ferritin, NL TIBC
Inc Ferritin, Inc/Dec Fe, Dec TIBC
Fe Restricted Erythropoiesis (infxn, inflam., CKD)
- Fe
- PRBCs
- EPO (CKD)
- Rx underlying
NL Smear
Acute Blood Loss
- Reverse anticoag
- PRBCs
- Protonix
- Octreotide
- Scope
↑ retic, ↑ indirect bili (T bili - direct), ↑ LDH, ↑ haptoglobin
Smear
Pan-cytopenia
BM hypo-cellularity
Aplastic Anemia
- HSCT
- CYP
- Irradiated PRBCs/ Plts
Dec Folate, + ETOH
Folate Deficiency
Folic Acid 1 mg PO qd, no ETOH
Dec B12 + paresthesia
B12 Deficiency
B12 1,000 mcg PO qd or IM qmo
Inc Lead Level
Lead Toxicity
- Avoid
- Prevent
- Chelation
- IVF
- Mon I/O
Target Cells on Smear
Thalassemia
Deferoxamine if ferritin > 800, PRBCs, low Fe
Sickle Cells
SCD
- O2
- 150 mL/kg/d
- PRBCs
- K+
- Folate
- Hydroxyura
Bite Cells
G6PD
- Folate 5 mg qd
- Avoid infxn, fava, ASA, nitrofurantoin
Schistocytes
Microangiopathic Hemolytic Anemia
PT, PTT, BUN/SCr, LFTs, BP
See Schistocytosis
Spherocytes
+ DAT
See Coombs
- DAT
Hereditary Spherocytosis

Spherocytes, Coombs Test

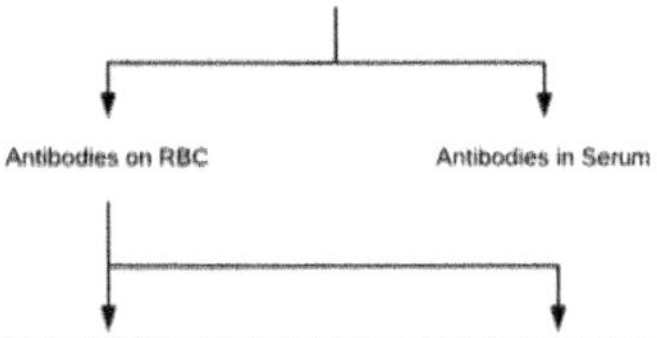

	Warm Antibody	Cold Antibody
Antigen	Rh Ag	i Ag
Direct Coombs Ab	IgG +/- C3	IgM, C3
Classification	Warm Antibody Autoimmune Hemolytic Anemia	Cold Antibody Immunohemolytic Anemia
Etiology	- SLE - CLL - Lymphoma - Meds (methyldopa, PCN [hapten], procainamide) - Idiopathic	- Quinidine (innocent bystander) - Lymphoma - Viral (IM, influenza) - Mycoplasma - Idiopathic cold hemagglutinin syndrome
Rx	Steroids, Danazol → Rituximab, splenectomy, immunosuppressants	CYP, chlorambucil → Rituximab, NO STEROIDS

Schistocytosis

Condition	Presentation	Diagnosis	Management
TTP (verotoxin, clopidogrel, pregnant Dxs, cyclosporin, tacromilus, cancer, mitomycin)	Neuro: HA, forgetful, tinnitus, weakness Renal: hematuria, AKI Other: Fever	Hemolytic anemia Thrombocytopenia Clotting factors not deficient	Plasmapheresis Plts contraindicated
HUS	Bloody diarrhea, AKI after uncooked meat (verotoxin from E. coli 0157:H7), no neuro changes or fever	↑ BUN/SCr + Hemoccult/ guaiac	Supportive care HD PRN
HELLP	Hemolytic anemia Elevated LFTs Low Plts 3rd Tmx/PP	Characteristic syndrome	- MgSO4 4-6 g IV load, 1-2 g/hr x24h (Sz prop) - Dexamethasone (C/S OB for dose) - Labetalol 20 mg IV, 40-80 q10min, nicardipine gtt
DIC	Involves clotting factors (unlike rest)	↑ PT/PTT	Support
Prosthetic Valve	Sx anemia	Schistocytes only!	Eval valve
Pre-eclampsia	>20 wks, BP >140/90, HA, AP	Proteinuria, BP elevated	Same as with HELLP

Sickle Cell Anemia

Normocytic anemia where HbA → HbS → Clumping & Infarction d/t beta globin chain point mutation, increased prevalence in African American population (but described in all races).

Crisis Triggers: Infxn, fever, dehydration, hypoxia, cold exposure, physical or emotional stress

Acute Pain Crisis:
- Diagnosis of exclusion
- O2 only if SpO2 < 90%, causes myelosuppression increasing transfusion requirements
- No IVF bolus unless true hypovolemia (LR > NS because a/w atelectasis [acute chest], hyperchloremic metabolic acidosis [promotes sickling], & concurrent opioids increase vascular leak & predisposes to pulmonary edema
- Maintenance IVF w/ ½ NS or D5 ½ NS if euvolemic
- Transfusion: avoid if hemodilution, avoid in uncomplicated (↑ viscosity of blood → vaso occlusion, acute chest, CVA), consider if Hgb $\leq$ 4 g/dL or symptomatic
- Manage hyperkalemia d/t hemolysis
- Abx if suspected infxn, treat as immunocompromised if febrile
- Analgesics: what worked in past? What do you take at home? Double home dose or hydromorphone 1-2 mg IV q15m → PCA OR MSO4 6-12 mg IV q15m → PCA + NSAID in ST if no renal Dz +/- gabapentin/pregabalin +/- ketamine 20 mg (or 0.1-0.35 mg/kg) over 2-5 min q30 min
- Folic acid 1 mg PO qd
- Hydroxyurea 15 mg PO qd, titrate by 5 mg/kg/d q12wk (max 35 mg/kg/d) – prevents future crisis, increases HbF, but needs f/u and monitoring
- No steroids, immunize, and educate on risk factors

Complications

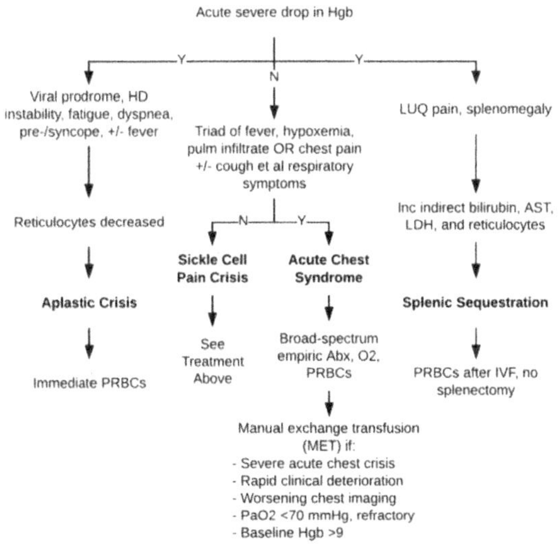

Blood Transfusion

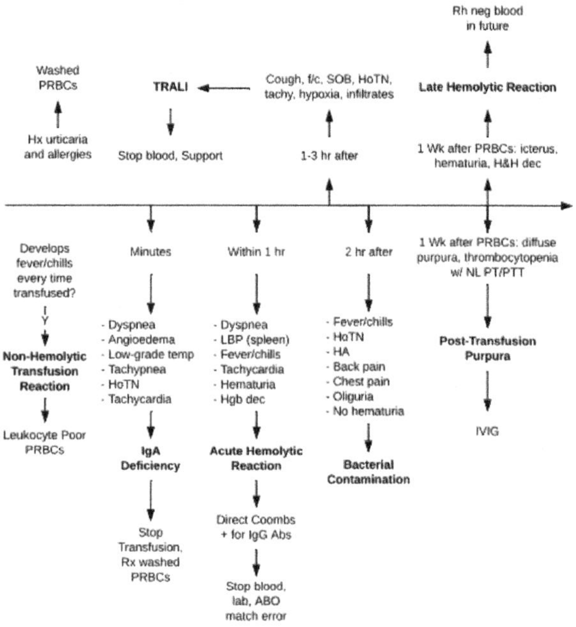

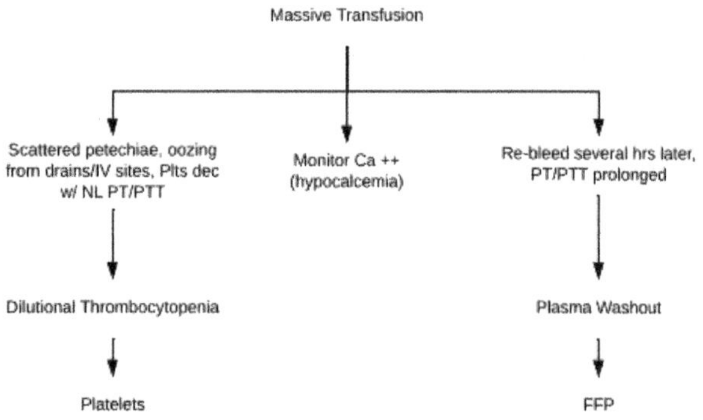

Thrombocytopenia

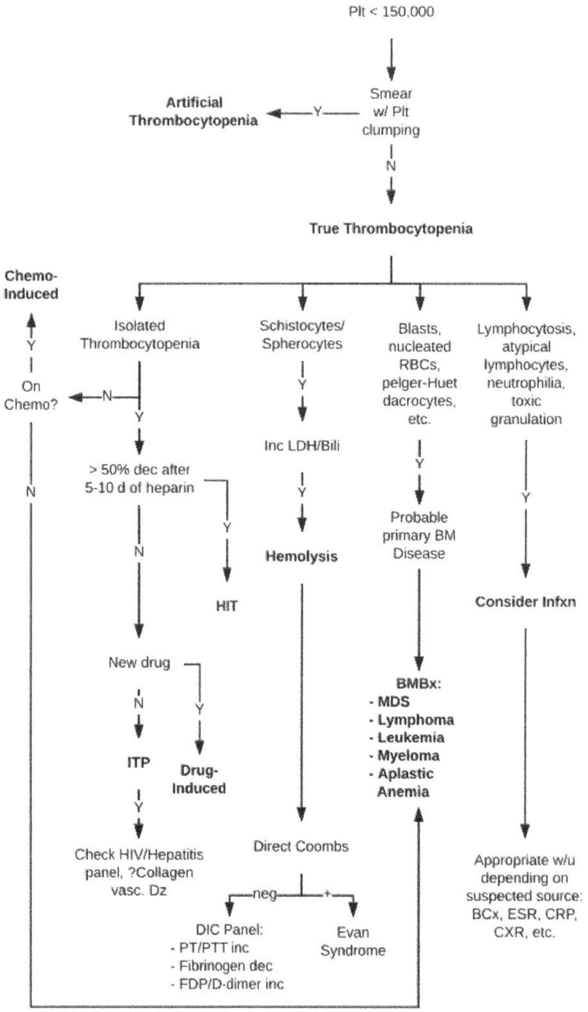

Bleeding Disorder, Normal Platelets

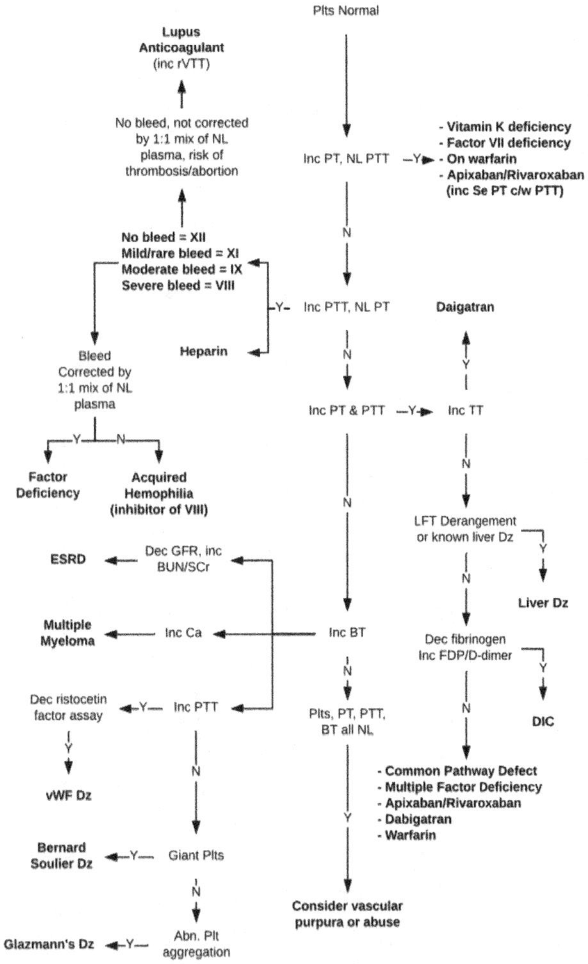

Coagulation Cascade

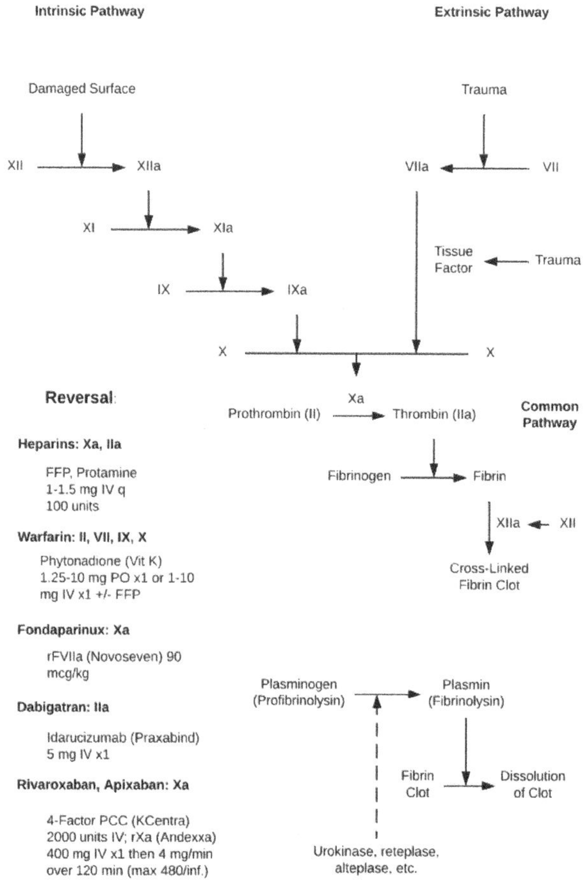

Reversal:

Heparins: Xa, IIa

FFP, Protamine
1-1.5 mg IV q
100 units

Warfarin: II, VII, IX, X

Phytonadione (Vit K)
1.25-10 mg PO x1 or 1-10
mg IV x1 +/- FFP

Fondaparinux: Xa

rFVIIa (Novoseven) 90
mcg/kg

Dabigatran: IIa

Idarucizumab (Praxabind)
5 mg IV x1

Rivaroxaban, Apixaban: Xa

4-Factor PCC (KCentra)
2000 units IV; rXa (Andexxa)
400 mg IV x1 then 4 mg/min
over 120 min (max 480/inf.)

Hypercoagulability/Thrombophilia

When to Test	Acquired Thrombophilia
- Idiopathic/recurrent VTE - VTE in < 50 y/o - Strong family Hx - Unusual site (cerebral, hepatic, mesenteric, renal) - Neonatal purpura fulminans - Warfarin-induced skin necrosis - Recurrent pregnancy loss 4-6 wks after acute event or D/C of anticoagulant/thrombolytic Rx vs. repeat when stable if checked acutely	- Immobilization (joint Sx, cast, bedrest) - Major surgery/trauma - Malignancies - Pregnancy - Oral contraceptives - Estrogen therapy - Antiphospholipid Ab syndrome - Heparin-induced thrombocytopenia - Paroxysmal nocturnal hemoglobinuria - Obesity - Smoking - Nephrotic syndrome

Screening	Reflex	Condition
PT/APTT	Lupus Anticoagulant Testing: DRVVT, PNP, and incubated APTT mixing study	Antiphospholipid Syndrome (APS)
Hexagonal phase phospholipid neutralization		
Anticardiolipin Ab assay	B2GP1 Ab Assay	
Protein C, Protein S, & Antithrombin functional assays	Protein C, Protein S, & Antithrombin functional assays	Protein C, Protein S, & Antithrombin Deficiency
CRP, Factor VIII, Fibrinogen		Elevated factor VIII, Dysfibrinogenemia
Activated Protein C resistance assay	Factor V Leiden SNP analysis	Factor V Leiden
Prothrombin G20210A SNP analysis		Prothrombin gene G20210A mutation
Homocysteine	MTHFR SNP Analysis	Hyperhomocysteinemia

Maintaining Hemostasis

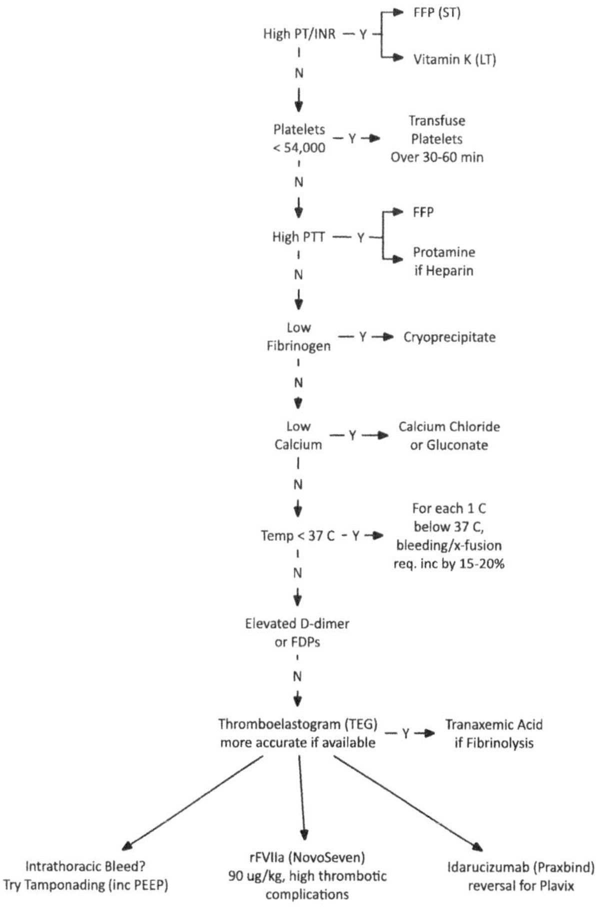

Venous Thromboembolism (VTE) & Pulmonary Embolism (PE)

Modified Wells Criteria:

- 3 Points
  - Clinical Sx of VTE
  - Other Dx less likely than PE
- 1.5 Points
  - Tachy (> 100)
  - Immobilization > 3 days
  - Previous VTE/PE
- 1 Point
  - Hemoptysis
  - Malignancy

> 4 points, further w/u warranted

Virchow's Triad

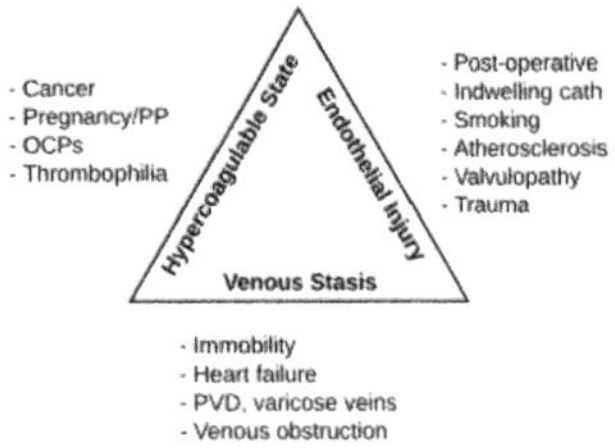

Diagnostics:

- Echo, RV strain/McConnell's sign
- CTA if SCr NL, VQ scan if AKI/CKD (inaccurate d/t central deposition if COPD)
- Venous ultrasound, non-compressible vein
- EKG, S1Q3T3 pattern
- ABG, isolated hypoxemia or resp. alkalosis
- D-dimer > 500, elevated BNP

Management:

- If RV strain +/- obstructive shock, consider tPA vs. thrombectomy
- If renal Dz, then Heparin gtt, otherwise enoxaparin 1 mg/kg q12h
- Bridge to warfarin:
  - Start 2-5 mg PO qd on day 1-2
  - Continue both until INR 2-3 (~5 days)
  - D/C LMWH/UFC 24h post therapeutic INR
  - Continue ≥ 12 wks (3 mo), longer if unprovoked
  - F/U INR OP
- Bridge to Apixaban
  - Start 10 mg PO BID x 7 days on day 2-3
  - D/C LMWH/UFC @ initiation
  - Then Apixaban 5 mg PO BID x 6-12 wks (6 months if PE)
  - More expensive, but no labs
- Can get OOB when > 48h of anticoagulation
- If unprovoked, will need indefinite anticoagulation
- If provoked, 6 month f/u scanning & hypercoagulable studies, if neg can D/C
- Prevent: leg exercise + hydration during flight + graduated knee-high compression stockings

VTE Prophylaxis (Enoxaparin):

- General: 40 mg SQ daily
- Knee surgery: 30 mg SQ BID
- Post-bariatric surgery: 40 mg SQ BID
- On prophylactic dose, needs LP: Hold x 12 h
- On treatment dose, needs LP: Hold x 24 h
- After LP, can restart in 4 h

Peripheral Smear

Finding	Correlation
Blister/bite cell	- G6PD Deficiency
Acanthocyte/Spurr Cell	- Liver Dz - Alcoholic Dz anemia
Echinocyte/Burr Cell	- Anemia of uremia
Howell Jolly Bodies	- Splenectomy and functional asplenia
Normoblast	- Severe hemolysis - Myelofibrosis
Polychromatophilia (Reticulocytes)	- Hemolysis - Blood loss - Bone marrow working
Schistocytes	- TTP - HUS - HELLP/Pre-eclampsia/fatty liver - DIC - Prosthetic valves
Spherocytes	- Hereditary spherocytosis - Autoimmune hemolytic anemia
Target Cells	- Thalassemia - Sickle cell disease - HbC - HbE - ETOH
Tear Drops	- Myeloid metaplasia w/ myelofibrosis - Thalassemia
Sideroblasts	- Myelodysplasia - Alcoholism - Vitamin B6 deficiency - Sideroblastic anemia

Oncology

Myelodysplastic Syndrome (MDS):

Pathogenesis: mutation/altered function of stem cell --> altered cell formation of hematopoietic cell lineage --> hypercellular BM with large # abn cells --> suppression of normal cell formation --> early death of these abnormal cells --> cytopenia

Presentation & diagnosis:

- Elderly patient
- With Dyspnea, weakness/fatigue
- Anemia +/- thrombocytopenia and/or leukopenia with **hyposegmented** PMNs
- Oval macrocytosis picture with dysfunctional platelets with megakaryocytes
- Refractory anemia with normocellular or hypocellular marrow
- BM: Marrow precursor dysplasia with ringed sideroblasts (survival 6 yrs)
- MDS with isolated 5q gene deletion (survival 12 yrs)
- > 10% blasts --> worse prognosis and may transform to AML (survival < 1 yr)

Management:

- < 55 yrs, allogenic BMT
- > 55 yrs, azacitidine (Vidaza) + supportive with blood transfusions, GCSF to ↑ WBCs
- EPO < 500, Rx EPO
- 5q gene deletion, lenalidomide (Revlimid)

Myelofibrosis:

- Other myeloproliferative disorders can "burn out" to myelofibrosis → extramedullary hematopoiesis → splenomegaly
- Smear: tear drop cells, nucleated RBCs, giant platelets
- BM aspiration: "dry tap"
- BMBx: ↑ collagen on reticulin stain, dysmorphic megakaryocytes
- Rx:
    - < 55 y/o, allogenic BMT, no splenectomy
    - > 55 y/o, supportive w/ blood transfusion +/- ruxolitinib

1 0 l—ALL—l 15 l—AML—l 35 l—CML—l 60 l—CLL—>

Acute Myelocytic Leukemia (AML):

- Young adult with superficial bleeds/infxns, leukocytosis, auer rods, blast cells, previous alkylating agents and topoisomerase inhibitors w/ previous myeloproliferative disorder (CML, myelodysplasia, or fibrosis)
- Infiltration of marrow w/ WBCs →
    - ↑ Immature WBCs (blast cells > 20% in smear and BM, infxns [aspergillosis, pseudomonas])
    - ↓ plts → superficial bleeds
    - ↓ Hgb → anemia, fatigue
- Myeloperoxidase stain + in M2 to M5, M3 (acute pro-myelocytic leukemia t(15,17) auer rods = good prognosis w/ differentiation)
- t(9,22) abr/bcl w/ previous cancers and multiple cytogenic abn = bad prog
- Rx:
    - < 50 y/o, allogenic BMT
    - > 50 y/o, ara-C (Cytarabine) and DNA (daunorubicin)
    - M3, all-trans retinoic acid (ATRA) + arsenic trioxide
        - Presents w/ low-grade fever, SOB, and BLE edema w/out CP/cough 1 wk after starting = ATRA differentiation syndrome, Rx dexamethasone

Chronic Myelocytic Leukemia (CML):

- ↑ WBCs > 50k, ↓ leukocyte alkaline phosphatase (LAP), Ph chromosome +, splenomegaly
- Dx: fluorescent in situ hybridization (FISH) for t(9,22) Ph chromosome or PCR analysis for the abl/bcr fusion gene
- 25%/yr transform → Blast crisis → AML (fever, night sweats, bone pain, blast cells) → Poor prognosis
- Rx:
  - < 50 y/o, imatinib
  - > 50 y/o, imatinib mesylate → tyrosine kinase inhibitor, alpha interferon, hydroxyurea, busulfan
  - Splenomegaly → early satiety, LUQ fullness

Acute Lymphocytic Leukemia (ALL):

- More difficult to treat in adults than children (90% remission in child)
- Pancytopenia w/ circulating blasts is hallmark (BMBx to confirm)
- Rx: chemo, BM x-plant, control Sx

Chronic Lymphocytic Leukemia (CLL):

- > 60 y/o with lymphocytosis, lymph nodes +, smudge cells, AIHA, infxns (very elevated WBCs = chronic; elevated blasts = acute)
- Lymphocytes (small, mature, smudge cells), hypogammaglobulinemia (recurrent infxns), autoantibodies (autoimmune hemolytic anemia)
- Lymphocytes express T cell marker CD 5 and B cell marker CD20 and CD23
- Rx:
  - Asymptomatic: No Rx
  - Symptomatic: Fludarabine, chlorambucil, rituximab
  - IVIG for infxns
  - Lymphocytosis alone = no Rx; Lymphocytosis + anemia, Hgb < 11 = treat; lymphocytosis + thrombocytopenia < 100k = treat

Non-Hodgkin's Lymphoma (NHL):

- Cause unknown, may have viral etiology
- Often presents with LAD
- Most common neoplasm between 20-40 y/o
- Less predictable pattern of spread than HL

Hodgkin's Lymphoma (HL):

- Cause is unknown
- More common in males, avg. 32 y/o
- Usually presents w/ cervical LAD and spreads in a predictable fashion along lymph node groups
- Characteristic Reed-Sternberg cells on BMBx differentiate from NHL

HL/NHL Dx:

- CT, MRI, PET to locate and stage
- Bx and histopathologic analysis confirms Dx
- Staging: Based on Bx of enlarges lymph nodes
  - I = Localized Dz to single node/group
  - II = > 1 node group, confined to one side of diaphragm
  - III = Nodes/spleen involved on both sides of diaphragm
  - IV = Liver/BM involvement

HL/NHL Management:

- Radiation, chemo, BM transplant

Multiple Myeloma (MM):

- Lytic lesions, bone pain, hypercalcemia, serum & protein urine "M" spike
- Marrow cytosis > 10%
- Plasma cells → osteoclasts → punched out lesions → hypercalcemia
- → Immunoglobulin (faulty IgG) → "M" spike in serum & urine (kidney failure), rouleaux formation of RBCs, ↑ ESR, plt dysfunction, infxns

Cancer Screening Recommendations

Cancer s/s: weight loss, fatigue, anorexia, anergia

		ACS		USPSTF	
Type	**Test**	**Age**	**Frequency**	**Age**	**Frequency**
Breast	Mammograms	40 & up	Yearly	50-74	Q other yr
	CBE	20-39	Q3 yrs		
	BSE	20 & up	"optional"		
Cervical	Pap smear	21-39	Q3 yrs	21-65	Q3 yrs
	Pap w/ HPV	30-65	Q5 yrs	21-65	Q5 yrs
Colorectal	FOBT	50+	Yearly	50-75	"Risk & benefits"
	Fecal Immuno-chemical test (FIT)		Yearly	50-75	" Risk vs benefits vary"
	Sigmoidoscopy		Q5 yrs		
	Colonoscopy		Q10 yrs		
	CT "virtual" colonography		Q5 yrs, f/u colon if +	"Insufficient evidence to assess risk vs. benefit"	
Lung	CXR, CT, PET, bronch	55-74; rec for fairly good health + 30 yr smoking + still smoking or quit w/in past 15 yrs		"Evidence insufficient to rec for or against screening in asymptomatic pts"	
Prostate	PSA, DRE Slow growing	> 50 y/o, > 45 y/o African American or men w/ family history		"Rec against PSA-based screening for prostate CA"	
Testicular	TSE/CSE	Include as regular part of physical exam		"Recommends against screening"	
Skin	Inspection	"Regular self- and provider- exams"		"Evidence insufficient to assess risk vs. benefit of whole-body exams"	

Pancreatic Cancer:

- Smoker, diabetic w/ cancer s/s w/ + Courvoisier's sign (painless palpable GB)
- CT with double line sign
- CA 19-9 +

Hepatocellular Carcinoma (HCC):

- Diarrhea, flushing, telangiectasia
- 5-HIAA > US liver (low Se)

Endocrinology

Diabetes Mellitus

	Type I	Type II
Patho	Autoimmune destruction of beta cells over months to years → absence of insulin	Gradual relative insulin deficiency (demand > supply) w/ reduced insulin sensitivity
Etio	Genetic: HLA DR haplotypes DR3 & 4 present in 95% pts, variation results in beta cell ID & destruction Environmental: Virii, toxins, breast feeding in 1st 6 mo protective	Obesity → adopokines → inhibition of TNF-a, 6, leptin, resistin et al. → interference w/ ICF signaling pathways Cushings, pheo, hyperthyroidism, insulinoma, antipsychotics
Pres	Polyuria (osmotic diuresis), thirst & blurred vision (hyperosmolar), wt loss (fluid voliume, ↓ muscle mass), dizziness/weakness/OH (volume, hypokalemia), paresthesia (neurotox)	Chronic skin infxns Candidal vaginitis (1st C/C in women) Visual disturbance d/t retinopathy Foot pain/infxn d/t peripheral neuropathy Sx DM I if more severe insulin def.
Comp	Diabetic Ketoacidosis (DKA)	Hyperglycemic Hyperosmolar Non-ketotic syndrome (HHNS)
Dx	Antibodies to glutamic acid decarboxylase (earliest) Islet cell antibodies (later) Ketones (urine/blood) Fasting blood glucose BUN/SCr >20:1 ?dehydration	***Metabolic syndrome*** – significant ↑ in cardiac Dz; 3+ of the following: - Waist circumference ≥ 40 inches (male) or ≥ 35 inches (female) - BP ≥ 130/85 - TG ≥ 150 - FBG ≥ 100 - HDL < 40 (M) or <50 (F) * HTN, BMI >25 + sedentary, >45 y/o → check FBG

Blood Glucose & HbA1c Analysis

	Normal	Prediabetes	Diabetes Mellitus
Fasting blood glucose (mg/dL), no caloric intake x 8 hours	< 100	100 – 125	≥ 126 x2 (microvascular risk)
2 h after glucose load (oral glucose tolerance test [OGT]) (mg/dL)	< 140	140 – 199	≥ 200
HbA1c (%), 120-day avg. glucose use	< 5.7	5.7 – 6.4	≥ 6.5
Symptoms & random glucose level (mg/dL)	N/A	N/A	≥ 200

Average Glucose per A1c = (28.7 x HbA1c) – 46.7 q1% ↓ HbA1c = 30 mg/dl ↓ BG

False ↑ HbA1c	False ↓ HbA1c
↓ RBC turnover (↓ reticulocytes)	↑ RBC turnover (↑ reticulocytes)
Hemoglobinopathies (d/t ↓ turnover; SCD, thalassemia, IDA, FDA, ↓ B12), ESKD (↓ EPO), asplenia (↑ RBC lifetime)	Hemolytic anemia, HIV, transfusion; Rx for IDA, FDA, ↓ B12

Management of Diabetes Mellitus

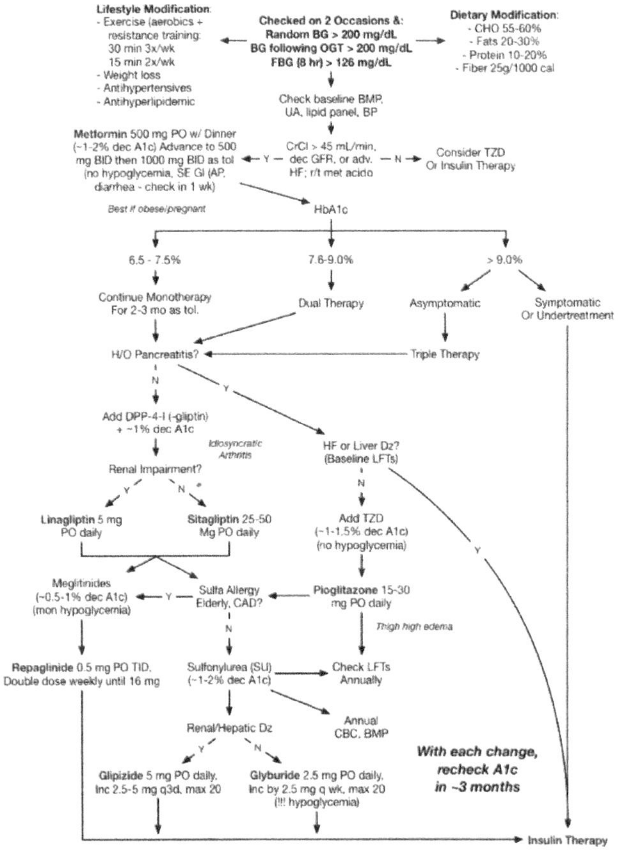

Insulin Therapy

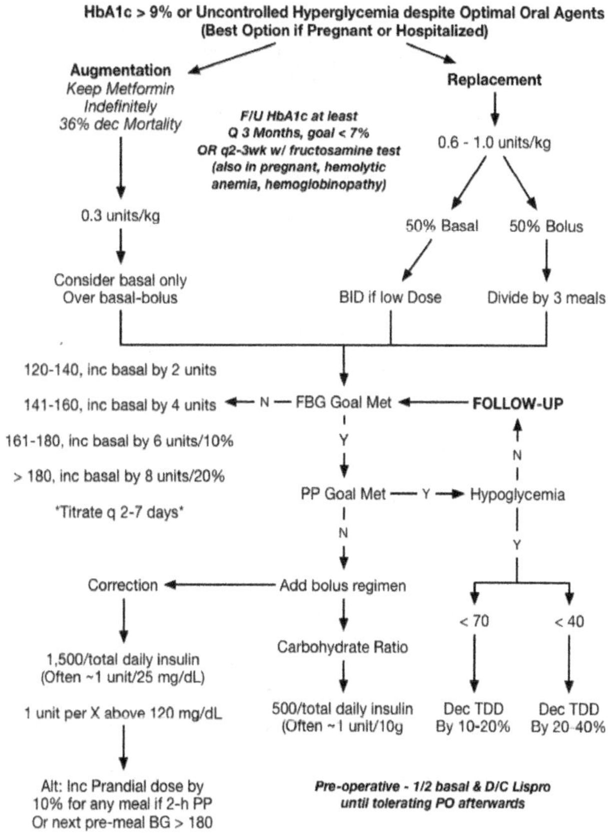

70/30 mix is cheapest! 24 hours SSI usage = BID dose

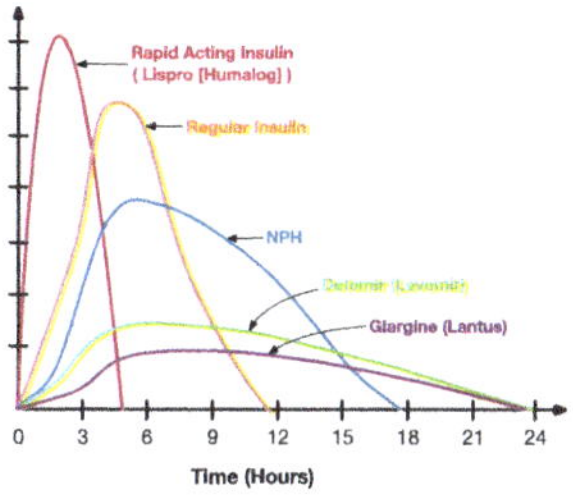

Drugs Causing Hyperglycemia

- Statins
- Beta blockers
- HCTZ
- Niacin
- Olanzapine
- Protease inhibitors
- Steroids

Analysis of Early Morning Hyperglycemia

Somogyi Effect:

- ***Somogyi = SO MOch insulin***
- Nocturnal hypoglycemia develops resulting in a surge of counter-regulatory hormones (Somogyi effect) which raises BG
- Presentation – hyperglycemia at 0800
- Diagnosis – hypoglycemia at 0300
- Treatment – Reduce/omit the HS dose of insulin

Nocturnal Hypoglycemia:

- **Wake up w/ HA**, fatigue, diaphoresis +/- nightmares
- Dx – check 3 am BG
- Rx – ↓ NPH OR move to HS OR change to LAI

Dawn Phenomenon:

- ***Dawn = Down insulin, BG rises w/ sun***
- Results when tissue becomes desensitized to insulin nocturnally (hormonal, ↑resistance)
- Leading cause of ↑ FBG
- Presentation – hyperglycemia at 0800; **wake up w/ HA**, fatigue, diaphoresis
- Diagnosis – hyperglycemia at 0300-0700 (BG progressively elevates throughout night)
- Treatment – add or ↑ HS insulin dose

Hyperglycemia vs. Hypoglycemia

Hyperglycemia	Hypoglycemia
Hot and Dry, Sugar High	Cold and Clammy, Eat some Candy
Parasympathetic	Sympathetic
Insulin vs. PO antidiabetic	Rule of 15

Hypoglycemia

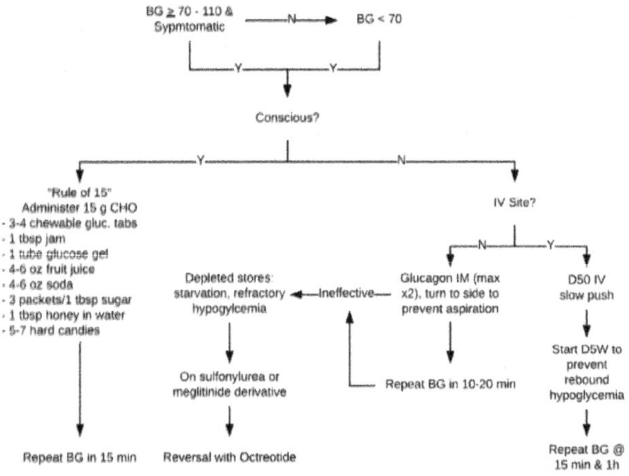

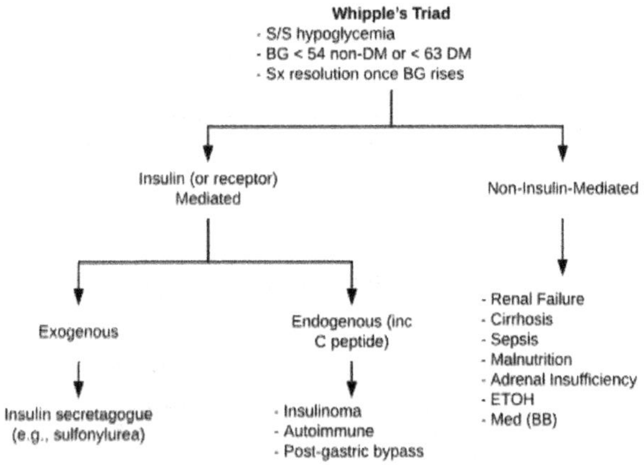

DKA vs. HHNS

Criterion	DKA			HHNS
	Mild	Moderate	Severe	
BG (mg/dL)	> 250	> 250	> 250	> 600
pH	7.25 – 7.3	7.0 – 7.24	< 7	> 7.3
HCO3- (mEq/L)	15 – 18	10 – < 15	< 10	> 15
Urine Ketones	+	+	+	Small
Serum Ketones	+	+	+	Small
SOsm (mOsm/kg)	Variable	Variable	Variable	> 300
Anion Gap	> 10	> 12	> 12	Variable
Mental Status	Alert	Alert/Drowsy	Stupor/Coma	Stupor/Coma

DKA Management Algorithm

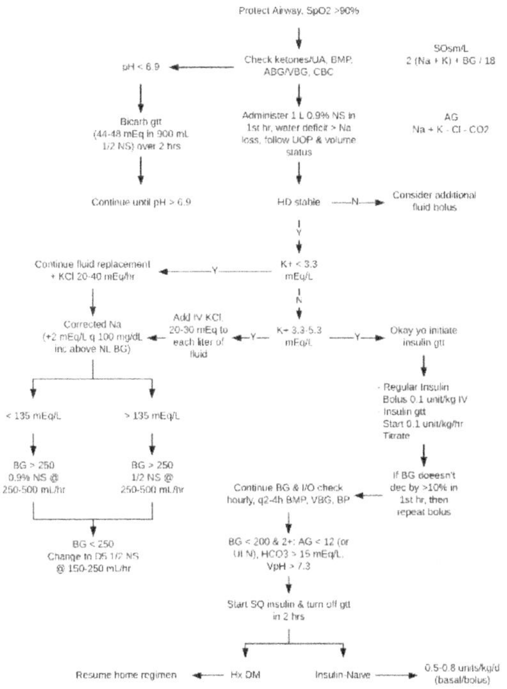

HHNS Management

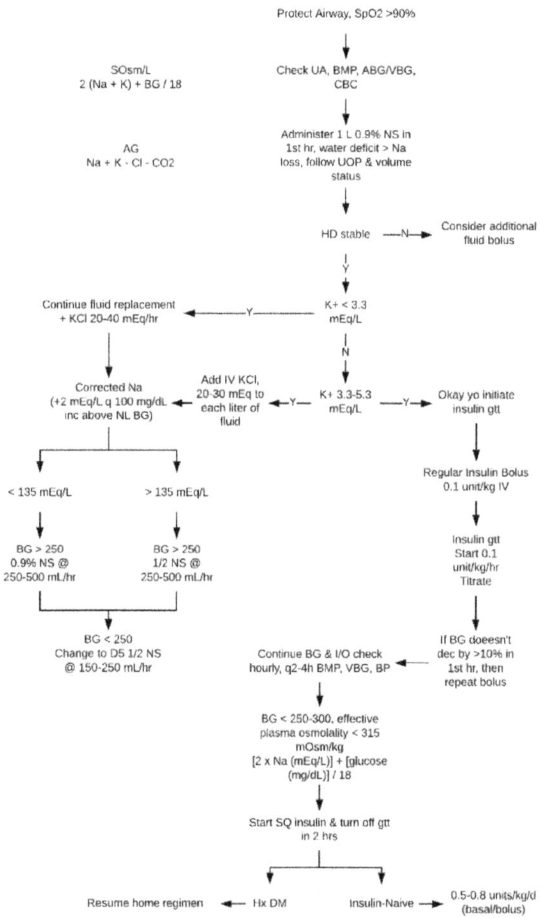

Alternative Transition from IV to SQ Insulin

Average Hourly Rate of IV Insulin			Dose of Basal Insulin			Dose of Scheduled Short/Rapid Insulin			Correction Scale
1	U/hr	=	8	U daily	And	2	AC/q6h	And	Very low dose
1.5	U/hr	=	12	U daily	And	3	AC/q6h	And	Very low dose
2	U/hr	=	16	U daily	And	4	AC/q6h	And	Very low dose
2.5	U/hr	=	20	U daily	And	5	AC/q6h	And	Very low dose
3	U/hr	=	24	U daily	And	6	AC/q6h	And	Very low dose
4	U/hr	=	32	U daily	And	8	AC/q6h	And	Very low dose
5	U/hr	=	40	U daily	And	10	AC/q6h	And	Low dose
6	U/hr	=	48	U daily	And	12	AC/q6h	And	Low dose
7	U/hr	=	56	U daily	And	14	AC/q6h	And	Low dose
8	U/hr	=	30	U BID	And	16	AC/q6h	And	Moderate dose
9	U/hr	=	36	U BID	And	18	AC/q6h	And	Moderate dose
10	U/hr	=	40	U BID	And	20	AC/q6h	And	Moderate dose

Determine average hourly rate of insulin (over past 8 h) and multiply by 24h to determine daily IV insulin requirement

Convert 2/3 (~ 70%) of daily IV insulin requirement to SQ insulin

- Give 50% as basal insulin, daily
- Give 50% as scheduled short/rapid acting insulin in divided doses
    - If enteral nutrition, divide by 4, give q6h
    - If enteral feeds stopped abruptly, start D10W at same rate as feedings and hold regular insulin
    - If pt eating, divide into 3 doses of rapid and give before meals
    - Hold if NPO

Determining SSI:

- Very low dose scale – on basal 0-32 units
- Low dose scale – on basal 33-56 units
- Moderate dose scale – on basal > 56 units

SSI Formula: (BG in mg/dL – 90) / (15)

If < 2 units/hr IV insulin, may not require transition to SQ insulin, consider low dose SSI and start basal only if uncontrolled with correction insulin.

Hyperthyroidism

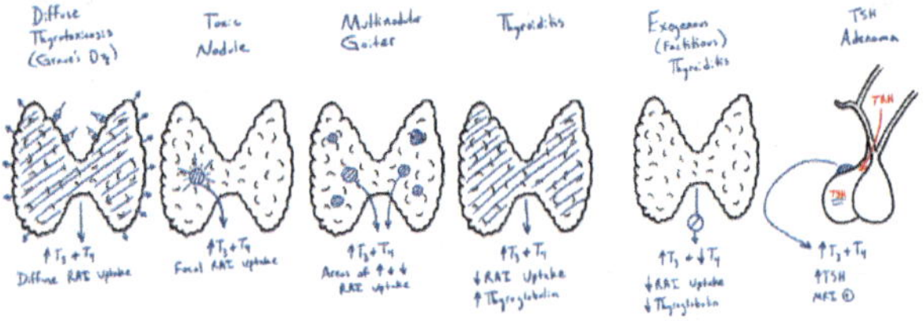

Management:

- Propylthiouracil (300 – 600 mg qd in 4 divided doses)
- Lugol's solution 2 – 3 gtts PO
  daily x 10 days to reduce vascularity of gland
- Propranolol (Inderal) 10 – 80 mg PO QID for symptom relief
- Radioactive iodine 131-1 to reduce goiter
- Thyroid surgery (must be euthyroid pre-op)
- Rx subacute thyroiditis w/ propranolol
- Small, frequent meals & VS/tele

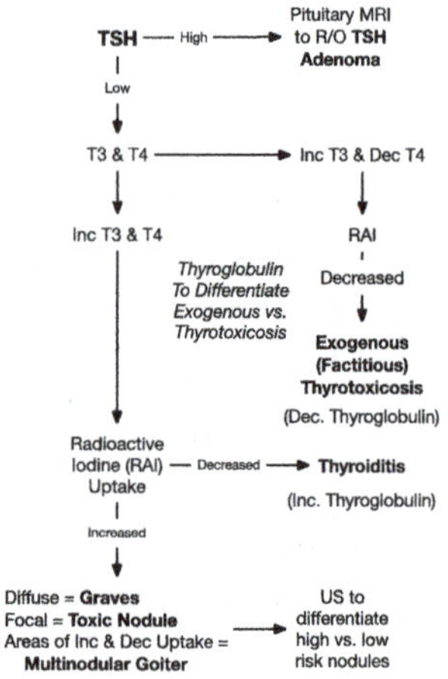

Thyroid Crisis/Storm

- Hypertensive urgency/emergency, hyperthermia, tachyarrhythmia (Afib), hyperreflexia
- ABCs, cooling measures
- Propylthiouracil 150 – 250 mg q4-6h (↓ by 45% w/in 24h vs. 10-35% w/ methimazole)
  - Lugol's solution 10 gtts TID OR
  - Sodium iodine 1 g slowly IV along +
  - Propranolol 0.5-2 mg IV q4h or 20-120 mg PO q6h (Esmolol gtt if HF) +
  - Hydrocortisone 50-100 mg q6h w/ rapid reduction as stimulation improves
  - +/- Digoxin if atrial fibrillation
  - Change to methimazole when stable
  - Avoid ASA! ↑ circulating thyroid hormone

Hypothyroidism

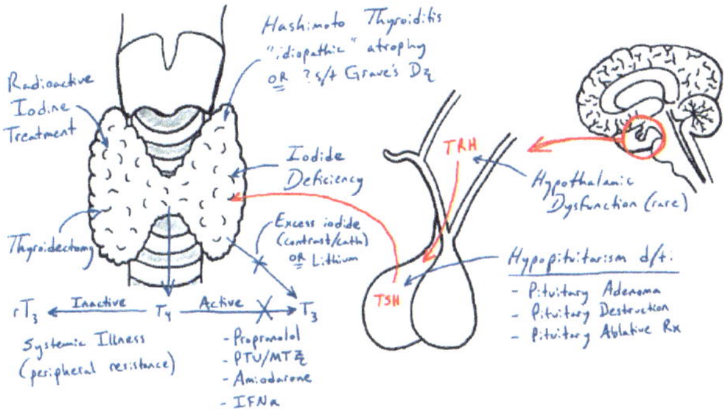

Levothyroxine (Synthroid) 25 mcg daily, can titrate by 25 mcg weekly until asymptomatic, repeat TSH 6 wks then q6-12 mo

- If > 60 y/o, start low & go slow

- Caution w/ HF, renal Dz (CV SE)

- Take on empty stomach, same time daily

Surgery for pituitary adenoma

T3 & T4

Low ↓

Check TSH

High ↙ → **Primary Hypothyroidism**

Low ↘ → **Hypopituitary Hypothyroidism** ↓ Pituitary MRI to R/O Adenoma

Myxedema Coma

- Presentation: Bradycardia, Hypothermia, Hypoactive DTRs, Hypoactive BS, Hypotension

- ABCs, IVF prn, vasopressors for BP support

- Levothyroxine (Synthroid) 200-400 mcg IV x1, then 50-100 mcg daily, then convert to PO

- Slow rewarming with blankets (not hyperthermia blankets) D/T risk for circulatory collapse

Hyperparathyroidism

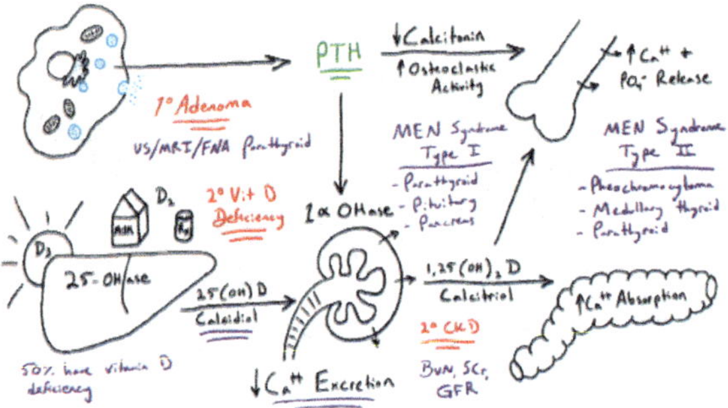

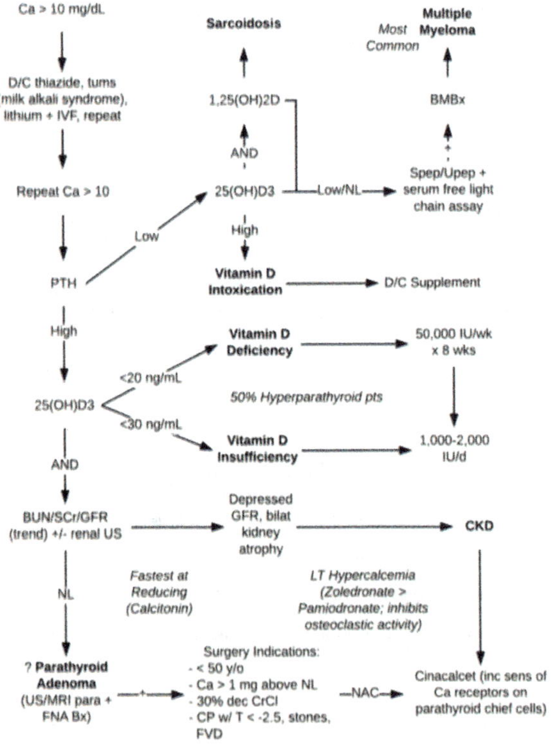

Hypoparathyroidism

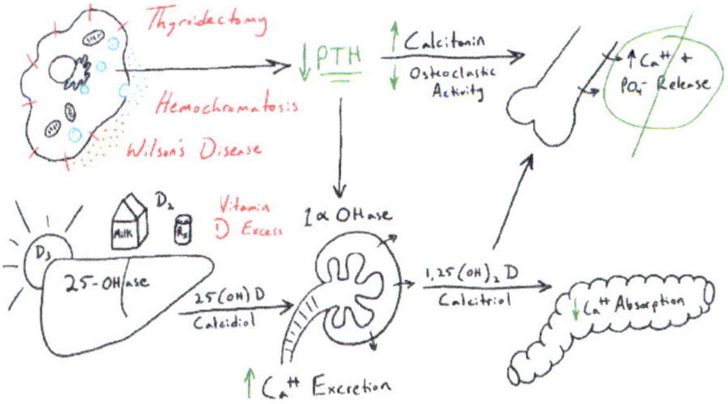

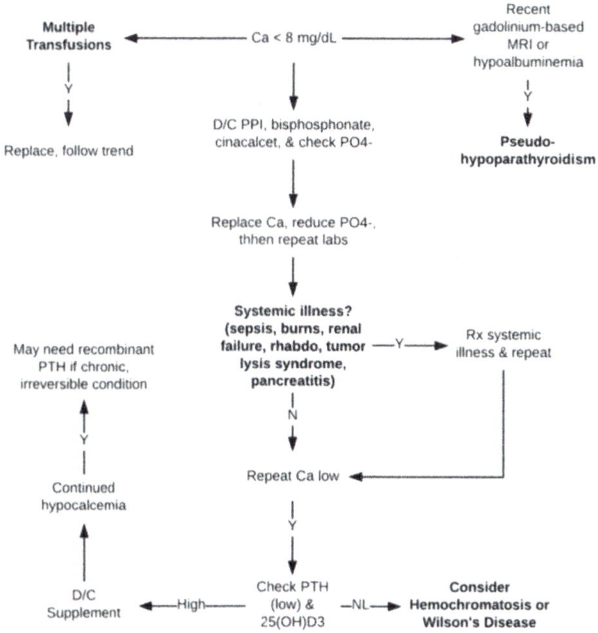

Adrenal Hormone Relationship

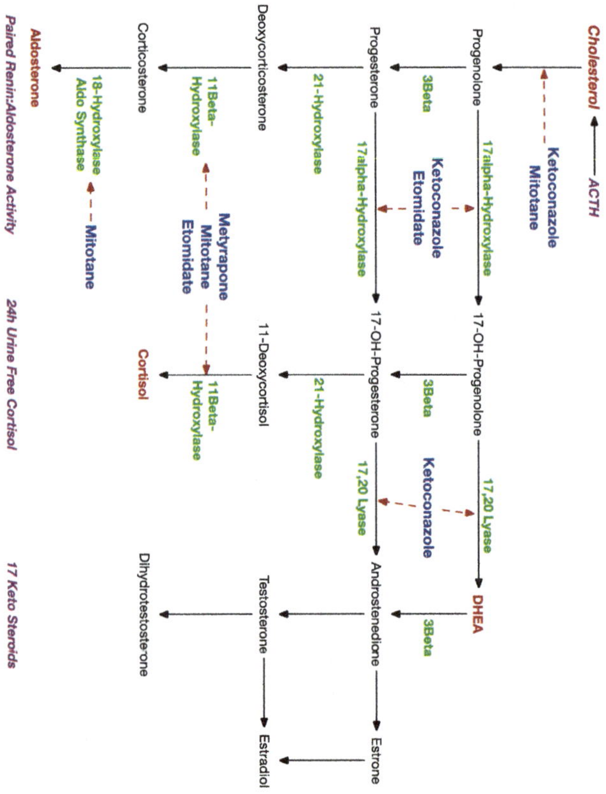

Cushing's Syndrome

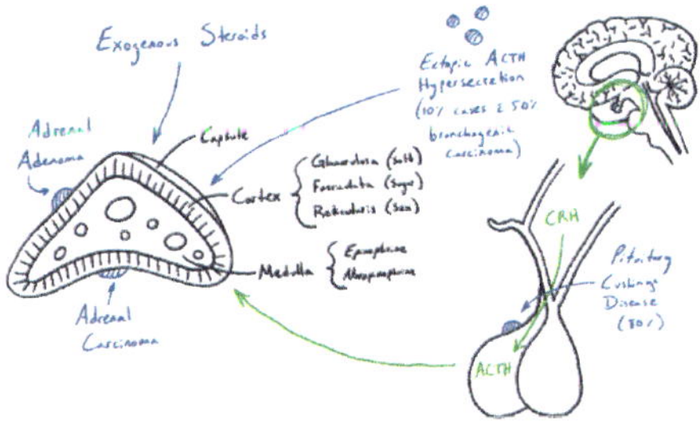

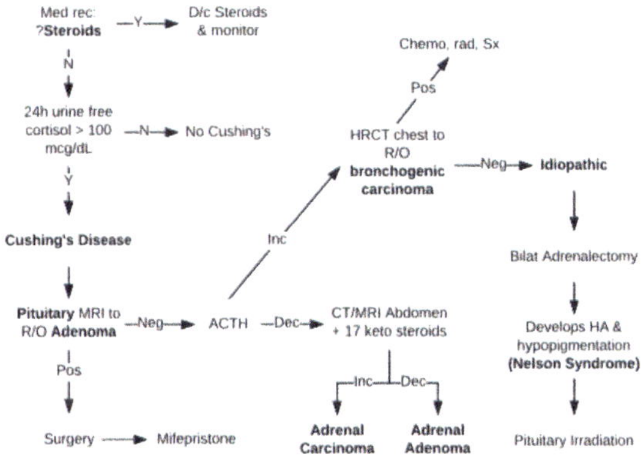

	Salt (aldosterone)	Sugar (cortisol)	Sex (androgens)
Sx	- Hypernatremia - Hypokalemia - Edema - HTN	- Hyperglycemia - Central obesity - Thin Skin - Purple striae - Moon face - Buffalo hump - Osteoporosis - Insomnia	- Masculinization of females - Amenorrhea - ↓ Libido - Impotence
Rx	- Low Na+ w/ high K+ diet (heart healthy) - K+ replacement - Antihypertensives - Diuretics (Spiro) - I/O and DWT - Cardiac monitoring	- Adrenal enzyme inhibitors (mitotane 6-12 mg/d [divided -], ketoconazole, metyrapone) - Exercise, PT - ?Insulin regimen	- Hormone replacement therapy
	Target etiology: surgical removal of adenoma; D/C causative meds		

Addison's Disease (Adrenocortical Insufficiency)

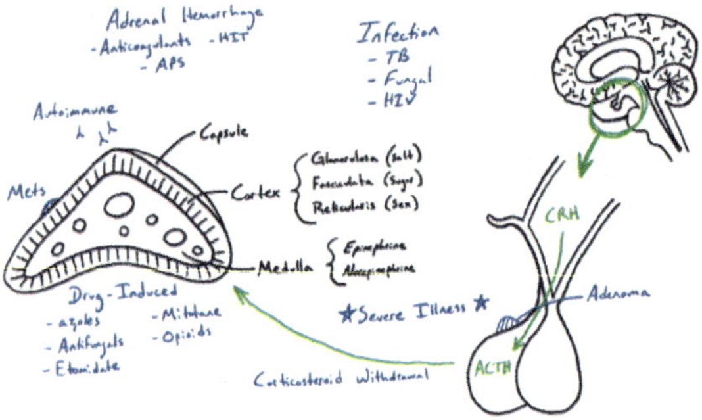

Able to do rapid ACTH stimulation test —N→ AM Cortisol (< 5 mcg/dL) + Plasma ACTH

Y ↓

1. Baseline Cortisol
2. Cosyntropin 250 mcg 0.25 mg IV x 1 dose
3. Cortisol @ 30 min
4. Cortisol @ 60 min

< 18 mcg/dL → **Primary Adrenal Failure**

> 18 mcg/dL → **Pituitary** → Pituitary MRI

AM Cortisol + Plasma ACTH:

>52 pg/mL → **Primary Adrenal Insufficiency**

<10 pg/mL → **Secondary Adrenal Insufficiency**

	Salt (aldosterone)	Sugar (cortisol)	Sex (androgens)
Sx	- Hyponatremia - Hyperkalemia - Dehydration - Hypotension - N/V/D	- Hypoglycemia - Fatigue - Weakness - Weight loss	- Amenorrhea - Loss of 2° sex characteristics
Rx	- NaCl tablets - 0.9% NaCl - ↑ Na+ intake - Fludrocortisone 0.05-0.2 mg/d - DWT and I/O - Monitor Lytes	- Hydrocortisone 15-25 mg PO daily (divided) - Alternatively: prednisolone 3-5 mg/d - Taper acute steroids - D5NS if hypoglycemic	- Prolonged corticosteroid use (controversial)

DI and SIADH Comparison

<table>
<tr><th>Diabetes Insipidus (DI)</th><th>Syndrome of Inappropriate ADH (SIADH)</th></tr>
<tr><td>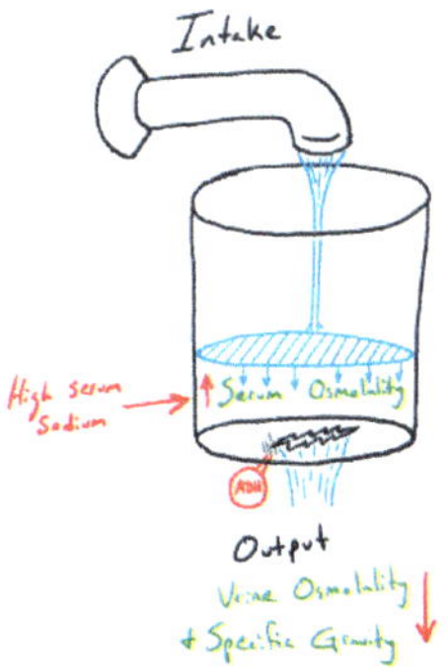
</td><td>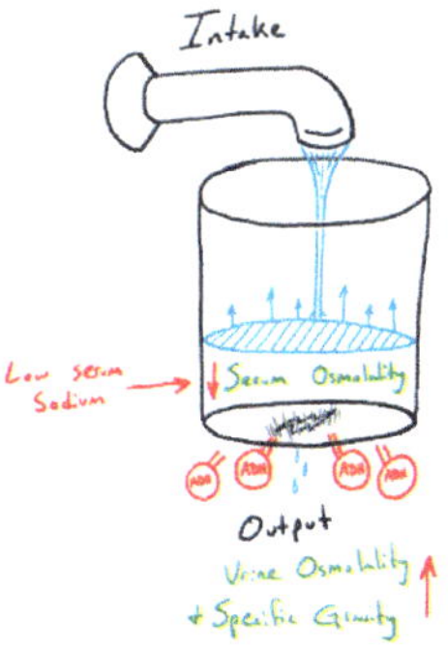
</td></tr>
<tr><td>"High and Dry"
↑ UOP
↑ Na (hypernatremia)
↑ SOsm
↓ USG
↓ UOsm
Dehydration
Water Loss
Hypotension</td><td>"Low and Wet"
↓ UOP
↓ Na (hyponatremia)
↓ SOsm
↑ USG
↑ UOsm
Fluid retention
Weight gain
Hypertension</td></tr>
<tr><td>- Congenital (X-linked, AD/AR)
- Hypercalcemia
- Hypokalemia
- Drugs (Lithium, Amphotericin B, nicotine, ETOH)
- Sickle cell anemia
- Amyloidosis
- Sjogren syndrome
- Sarcoidosis
- Fanconi Syndrome
- HIV infxn</td><td>- Post-operation
- Pituitary adenoma
- Infxn (meningitis)
- Lymphoma
- Idiopathic</td></tr>
</table>

Orthopedics & Rheumatology

Neck Pain

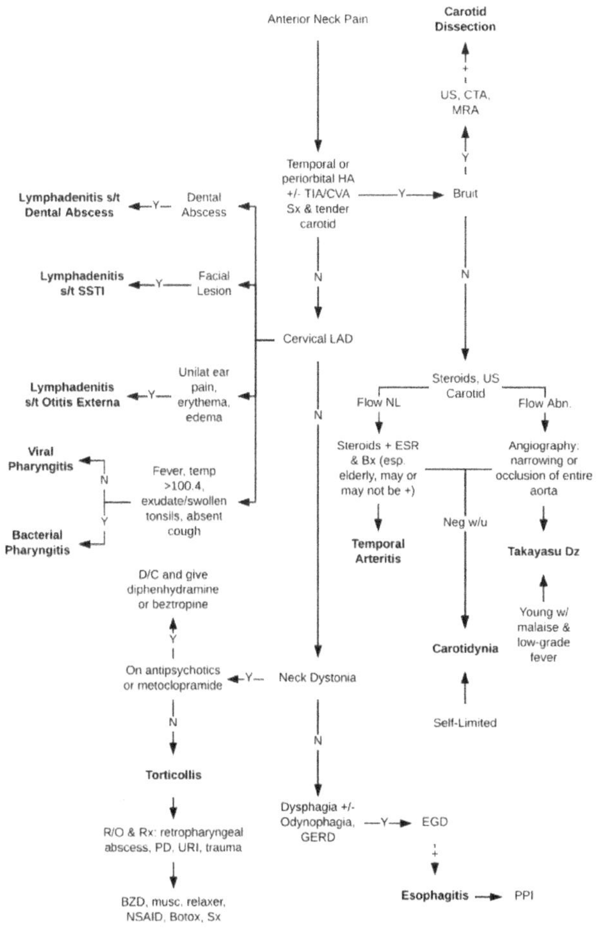
Anterior Neck Pain
Carotid Dissection
+
US, CTA, MRA
Y
Temporal or periorbital HA +/- TIA/CVA Sx & tender carotid
Y
Bruit
Lymphadenitis s/t Dental Abscess
Y
Dental Abscess
N
N
Lymphadenitis s/t SSTI
Y
Facial Lesion
Cervical LAD
Unilat ear pain, erythema, edema
Lymphadenitis s/t Otitis Externa
Y
N
Steroids, US Carotid
Flow NL
Flow Abn.
Steroids + ESR & Bx (esp. elderly, may or may not be +)
Angiography: narrowing or occlusion of entire aorta
Viral Pharyngitis
N
Fever, temp >100.4, exudate/swollen tonsils, absent cough
Y
Bacterial Pharyngitis
Neg w/u
Temporal Arteritis
Takayasu Dz
D/C and give diphenhydramine or beztropine
Y
Young w/ malaise & low-grade fever
Carotidynia
On antipsychotics or metoclopramide
Y
Neck Dystonia
Self-Limited
N
N
Torticollis
Dysphagia +/- Odynophagia, GERD
Y
EGD
R/O & Rx: retropharyngeal abscess, PD, URI, trauma
+
Esophagitis
PPI
BZD, musc. relaxer, NSAID, Botox, Sx

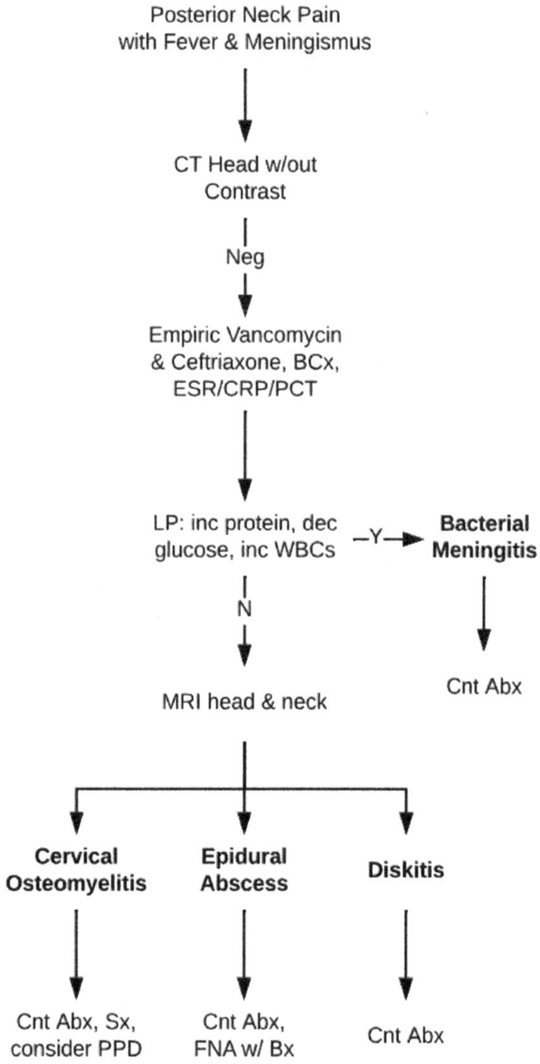
Posterior Neck Pain
with Fever & Meningismus
CT Head w/out
Contrast
Neg
Empiric Vancomycin
& Ceftriaxone, BCx,
ESR/CRP/PCT
LP: inc protein, dec
glucose, inc WBCs
Y
Bacterial
Meningitis
Cnt Abx
N
MRI head & neck
Cervical
Osteomyelitis
Epidural
Abscess
Diskitis
Cnt Abx, Sx,
consider PPD
Cnt Abx,
FNA w/ Bx
Cnt Abx

Posterior Neck Pain

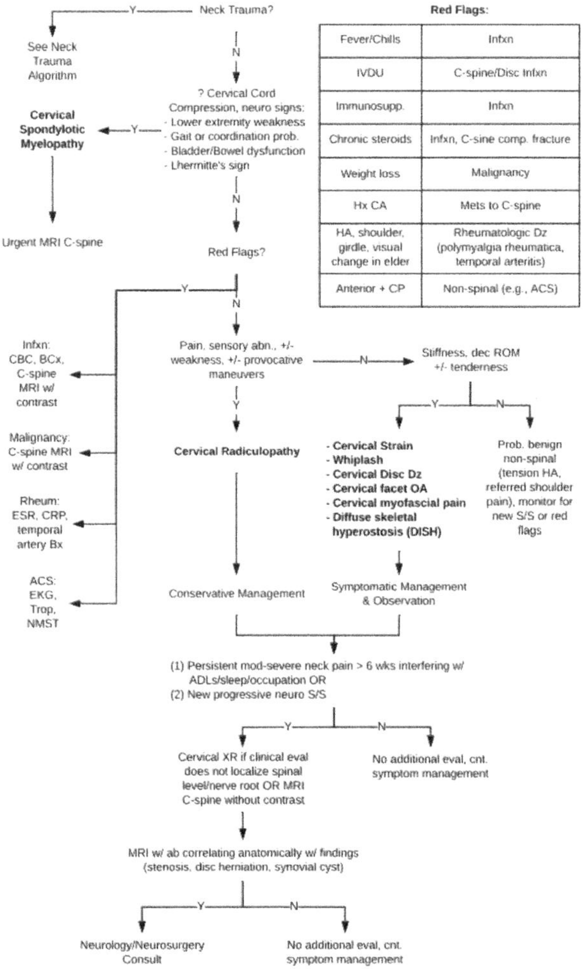

Red Flags:

Fever/Chills	Infxn
IVDU	C-spine/Disc Infxn
Immunosupp.	Infxn
Chronic steroids	Infxn, C-sine comp. fracture
Weight loss	Malignancy
Hx CA	Mets to C-spine
HA, shoulder, girdle, visual change in elder	Rheumatologic Dz (polymyalgia rheumatica, temporal arteritis)
Anterior + CP	Non-spinal (e.g., ACS)

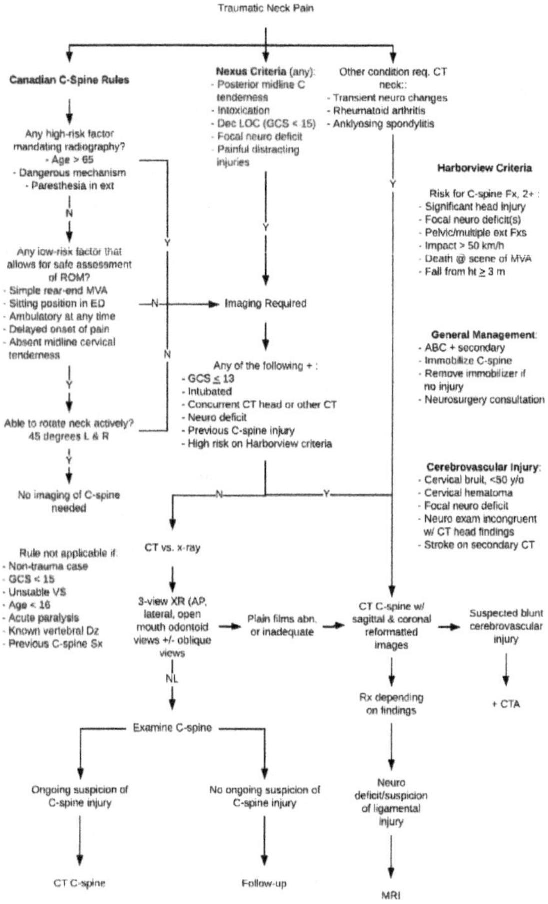
Traumatic Neck Pain
Canadian C-Spine Rules
Any high-risk factor mandating radiography?
- Age > 65
- Dangerous mechanism
- Paresthesia in ext
N
Y
Any low-risk factor that allows for safe assessment of ROM?
- Simple rear-end MVA
- Sitting position in ED
- Ambulatory at any time
- Delayed onset of pain
- Absent midline cervical tenderness
N
Y
Able to rotate neck actively? 45 degrees L & R
N
Y
No imaging of C-spine needed
Rule not applicable if:
- Non-trauma case
- GCS < 15
- Unstable VS
- Age < 16
- Acute paralysis
- Known vertebral Dz
- Previous C-spine Sx
Nexus Criteria (any):
- Posterior midline C tenderness
- Intoxication
- Dec LOC (GCS < 15)
- Focal neuro deficit
- Painful distracting injuries
Y
Imaging Required
Any of the following + :
- GCS ≤ 13
- Intubated
- Concurrent CT head or other CT
- Neuro deficit
- Previous C-spine injury
- High risk on Harborview criteria
N
Y
CT vs. x-ray
3-view XR (AP, lateral, open mouth odontoid views +/- oblique views
NL
Plain films abn. or inadequate
Examine C-spine
Ongoing suspicion of C-spine injury
CT C-spine
No ongoing suspicion of C-spine injury
Follow-up
Other condition req. CT neck::
- Transient neuro changes
- Rheumatoid arthritis
- Anklyosing spondylitis
Y
CT C-spine w/ sagittal & coronal reformatted images
Rx depending on findings
Neuro deficit/suspicion of ligamental injury
MRI
Suspected blunt cerebrovascular injury
+ CTA
Harborview Criteria
Risk for C-spine Fx, 2+ :
- Significant head injury
- Focal neuro deficit(s)
- Pelvic/multiple ext Fxs
- Impact > 50 km/h
- Death @ scene of MVA
- Fall from ht ≥ 3 m
General Management:
- ABC + secondary
- Immobilize C-spine
- Remove immobilizer if no injury
- Neurosurgery consultation
Cerebrovascular Injury:
- Cervical bruit, <50 y/o
- Cervical hematoma
- Focal neuro deficit
- Neuro exam incongruent w/ CT head findings
- Stroke on secondary CT

Shoulder Pain

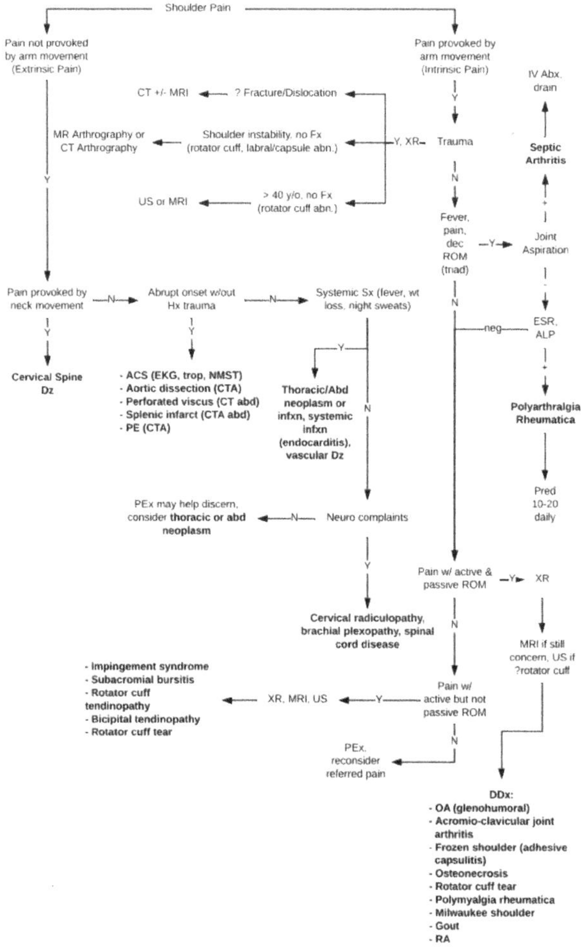

Forearm/Elbow Pain

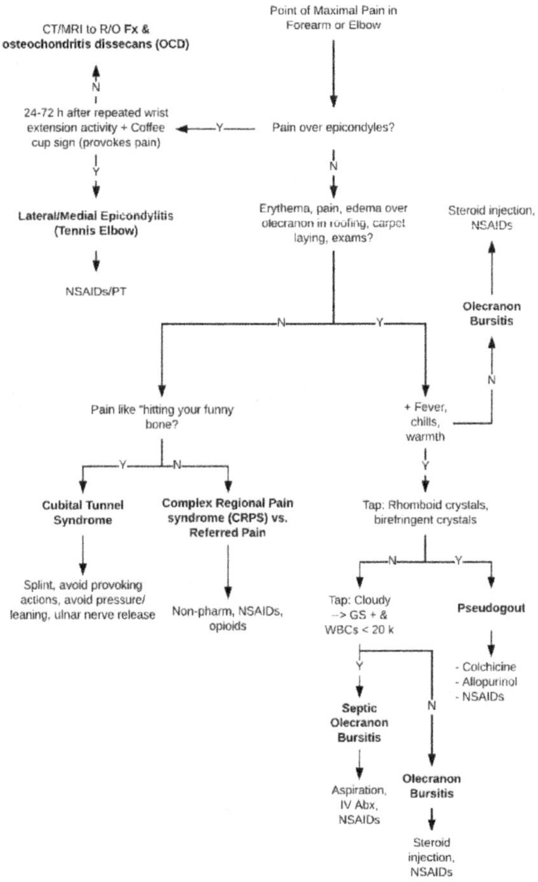

Wrist/Hand Pain

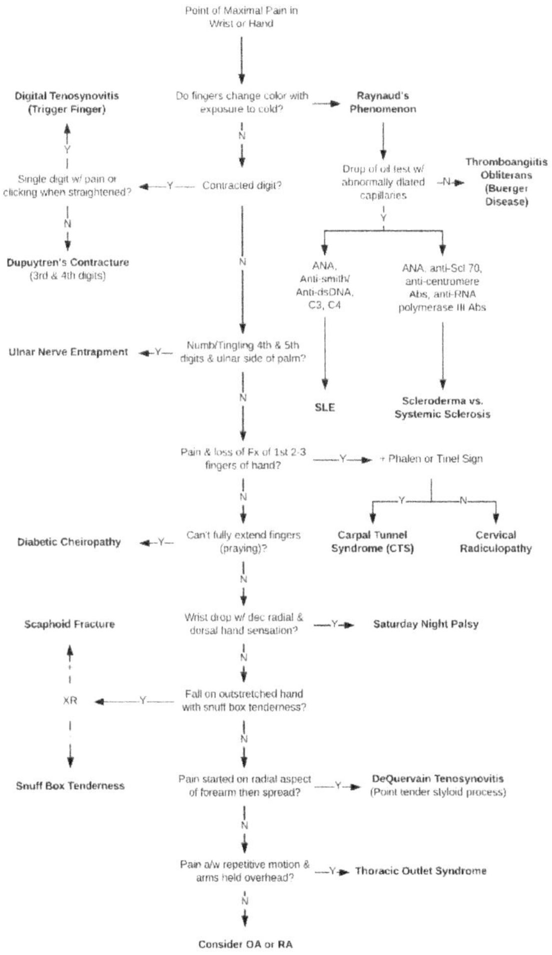

Low Back Pain

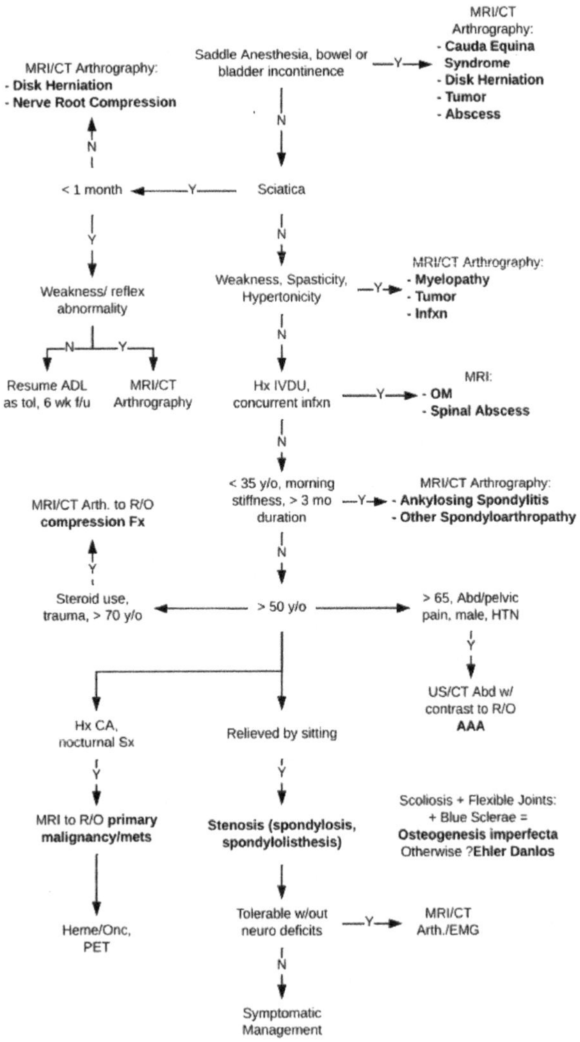

Buttock Pain

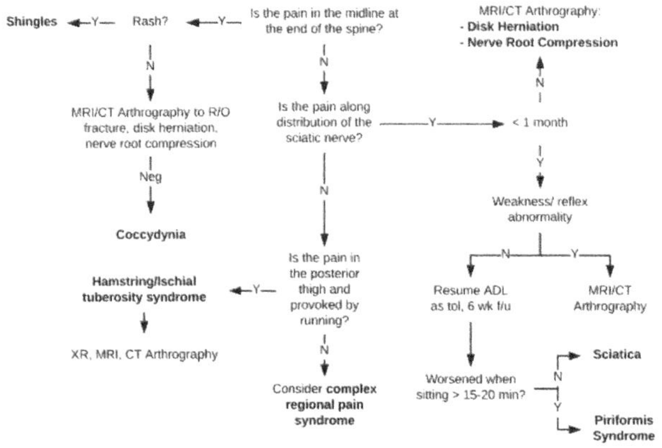

Thigh Pain

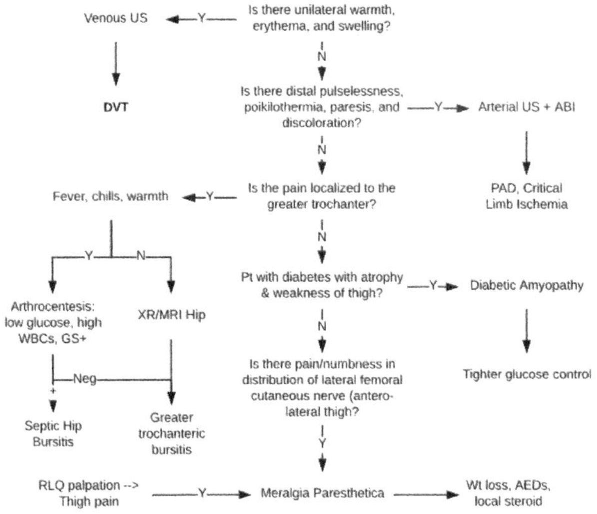

Anterior Hip Pain

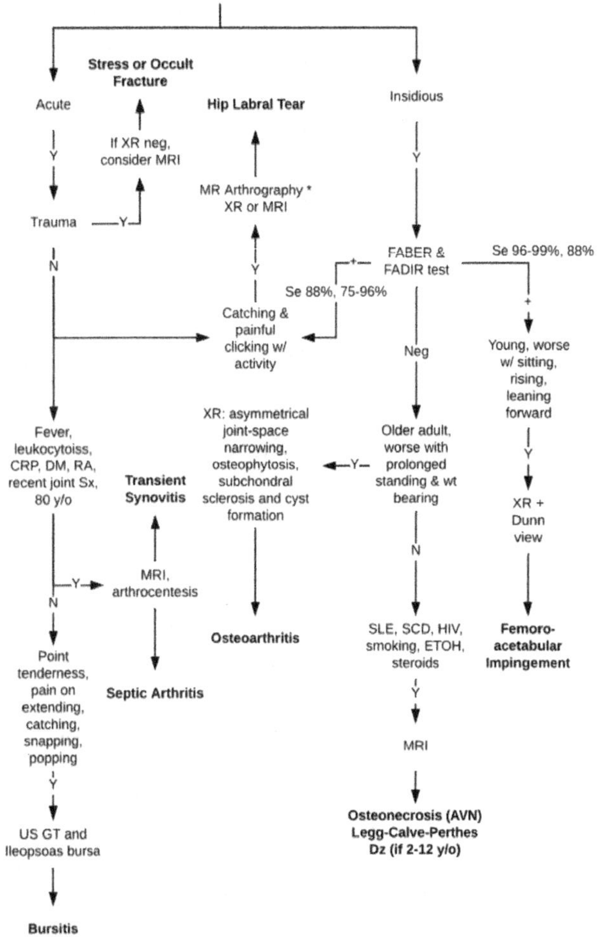

Knee Pain

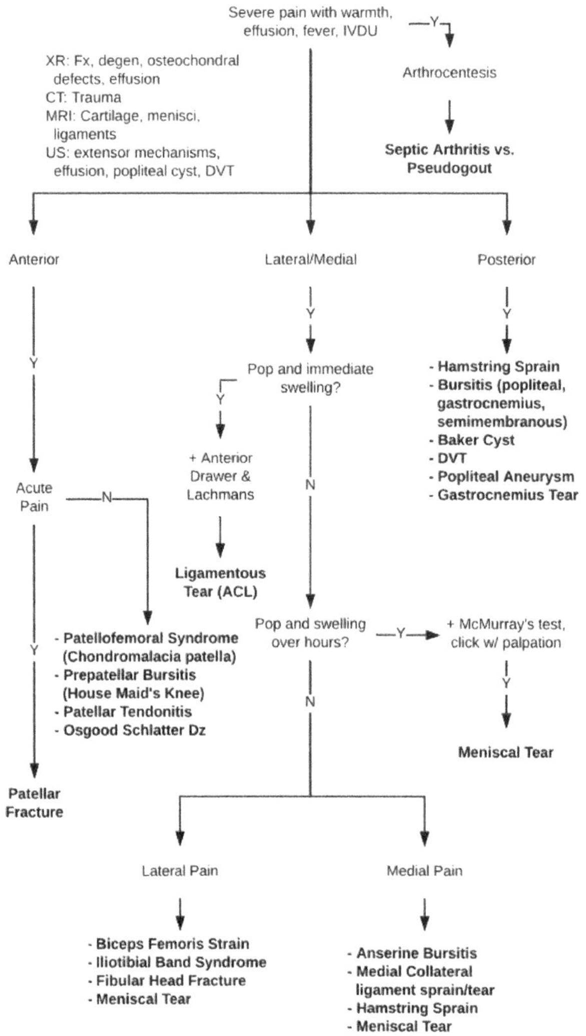

Severe pain with warmth, effusion, fever, IVDU
Y
Arthrocentesis
Septic Arthritis vs. Pseudogout
XR: Fx, degen, osteochondral defects, effusion
CT: Trauma
MRI: Cartilage, menisci, ligaments
US: extensor mechanisms, effusion, popliteal cyst, DVT
Anterior
Lateral/Medial
Posterior
Y
Y
Y
- Hamstring Sprain
- Bursitis (popliteal, gastrocnemius, semimembranous)
- Baker Cyst
- DVT
- Popliteal Aneurysm
- Gastrocnemius Tear
Pop and immediate swelling?
Y
+ Anterior Drawer & Lachmans
Ligamentous Tear (ACL)
N
Acute Pain
N
Y
- Patellofemoral Syndrome (Chondromalacia patella)
- Prepatellar Bursitis (House Maid's Knee)
- Patellar Tendonitis
- Osgood Schlatter Dz
Patellar Fracture
Pop and swelling over hours?
Y
+ McMurray's test, click w/ palpation
Y
Meniscal Tear
N
Lateral Pain
Medial Pain
- Biceps Femoris Strain
- Iliotibial Band Syndrome
- Fibular Head Fracture
- Meniscal Tear
- Anserine Bursitis
- Medial Collateral ligament sprain/tear
- Hamstring Sprain
- Meniscal Tear

Ankle Pain

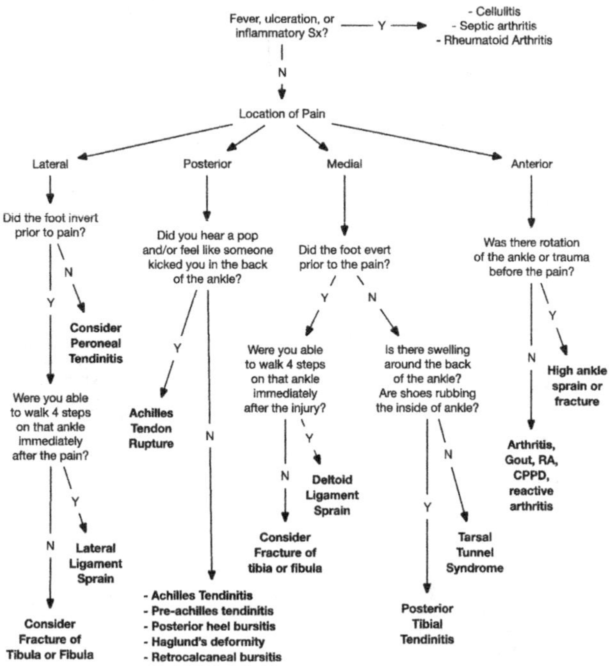
Fever, ulceration, or inflammatory Sx?
Y
- Cellulitis
- Septic arthritis
- Rheumatoid Arthritis
N
Location of Pain
Lateral
Posterior
Medial
Anterior
Did the foot invert prior to pain?
N
Y
Consider Peroneal Tendinitis
Were you able to walk 4 steps on that ankle immediately after the pain?
Y
Lateral Ligament Sprain
N
Consider Fracture of Tibula or Fibula
Did you hear a pop and/or feel like someone kicked you in the back of the ankle?
Y
Achilles Tendon Rupture
N
- Achilles Tendinitis
- Pre-achilles tendinitis
- Posterior heel bursitis
- Haglund's deformity
- Retrocalcaneal bursitis
Did the foot evert prior to the pain?
Y
N
Were you able to walk 4 steps on that ankle immediately after the injury?
Y
Deltoid Ligament Sprain
N
Consider Fracture of tibia or fibula
Is there swelling around the back of the ankle? Are shoes rubbing the inside of ankle?
N
Tarsal Tunnel Syndrome
Y
Posterior Tibial Tendinitis
Was there rotation of the ankle or trauma before the pain?
Y
High ankle sprain or fracture
N
Arthritis, Gout, RA, CPPD, reactive arthritis

Foot Pain

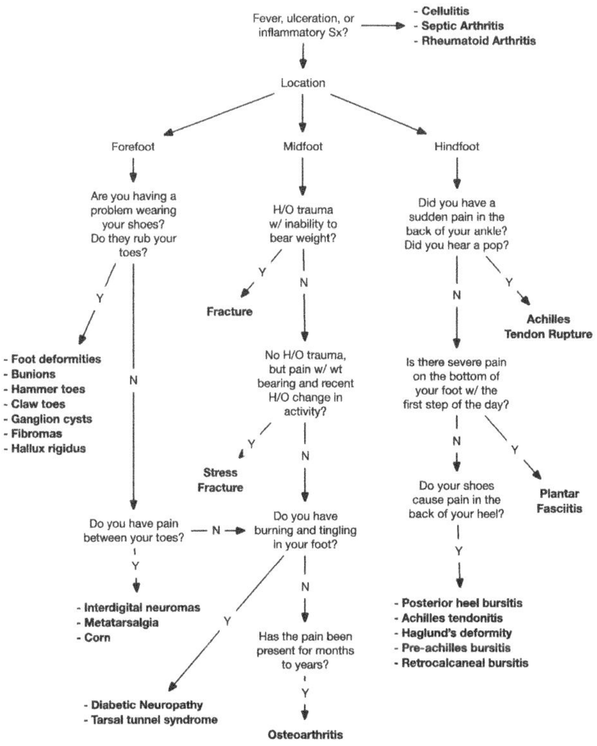

Fever, ulceration, or inflammatory Sx?
- Cellulitis
- Septic Arthritis
- Rheumatoid Arthritis
Location
Forefoot
Midfoot
Hindfoot
Are you having a problem wearing your shoes? Do they rub your toes?
Y
N
- Foot deformities
- Bunions
- Hammer toes
- Claw toes
- Ganglion cysts
- Fibromas
- Hallux rigidus
Do you have pain between your toes?
Y
N
- Interdigital neuromas
- Metatarsalgia
- Corn
H/O trauma w/ inability to bear weight?
Y
N
Fracture
No H/O trauma, but pain w/ wt bearing and recent H/O change in activity?
Y
N
Stress Fracture
Do you have burning and tingling in your foot?
Y
N
- Diabetic Neuropathy
- Tarsal tunnel syndrome
Has the pain been present for months to years?
Y
Osteoarthritis
Did you have a sudden pain in the back of your ankle? Did you hear a pop?
Y
N
Achilles Tendon Rupture
Is there severe pain on the bottom of your foot w/ the first step of the day?
Y
N
Plantar Fasciitis
Do your shoes cause pain in the back of your heel?
Y
- Posterior heel bursitis
- Achilles tendonitis
- Haglund's deformity
- Pre-achilles bursitis
- Retrocalcaneal bursitis

Polyarthritis

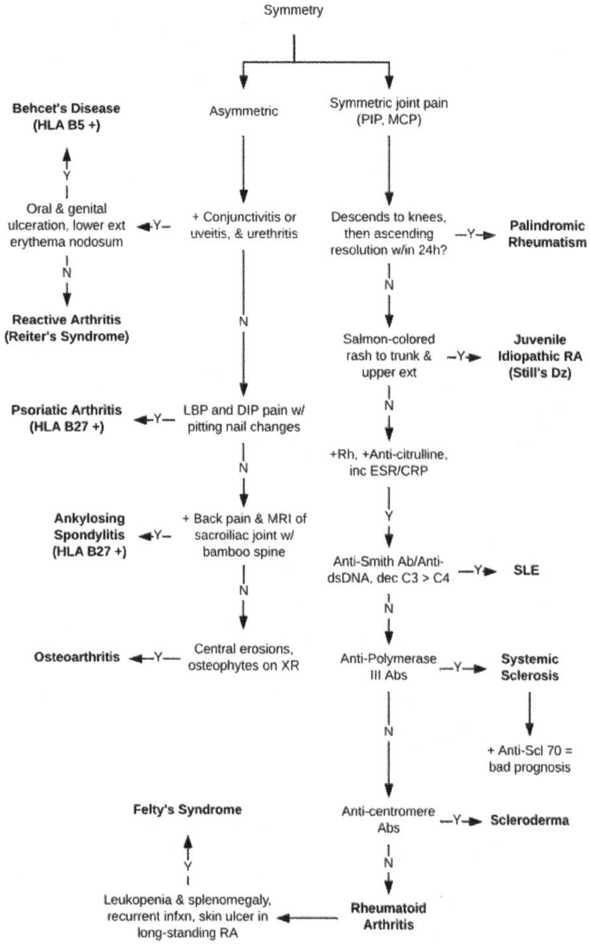

Arthrocentesis

Dz	Color	Clarity	WBCs	PMNs	Crystals	GS/Cx
Normal	Clear	Transparent	< 200	< 25%	None	-
Non-Inflammatory						
General	Yellow	Transparent	0-2000	< 25%	None	-
OA	Yellow	Clear	~ 700	~ 15%	None	-
Traumatic Arthritis	Straw	Cloudy	~ 1000	~ 25%	None	-
Inflammatory						
General	Yellow	Translucent-opaque	> 2000	≥ 50%	+/-	-
SLE	Straw	Clear	~ 2000	~ 30%	None	-
RF	Yellow	Slightly cloudy	~14,000	~ 50%	None	-
Pseudo-gout	Yellow	Cloudy	~15,000	~ 70%	Ca Pyro-phosphate, Rhomboid, +birefringent	-
Gout	Yellow to Milky	Cloudy	~20,000	~70%	Mono-Na Urate	-
RA	Yellow to green	Cloudy	~20,000	~70%	None	-
Infective						
General	Yellow	Opaque	> 20k	≥ 75%	None	+
Septic Arthritis	Yellow	Cloudy	~20,000	~60%	None	+
TB Arthritis	Grey or bloody	Turbid	~90,000	~90%	None	+
Hemorrhagic						
Hemorr-hagic	Red	Bloody	Var	50-75%	None	-

Psychiatry

Diagnostic Criteria by Symptom Duration

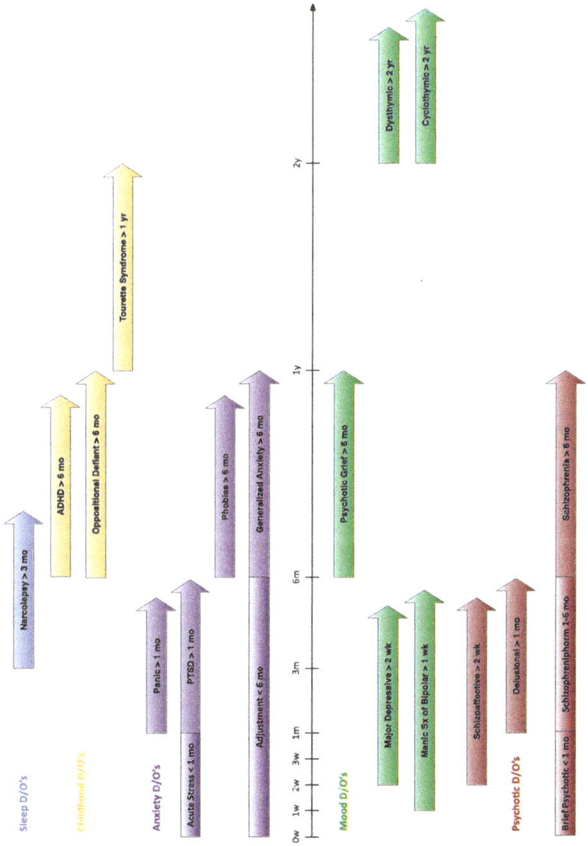

Delusions

Delusion of control:

- Another person, group of people, or external force controls one's thoughts, feelings, impulses, or behavior
- **Thought broadcasting**: belief that the affected person's thoughts are heard aloud
- **Thought insertion**: belief that an outside force, person, or group of people inserts thoughts
- **Thought withdrawal**: belief that an outside force, person, or group of people is removing or extracting a person's thoughts

Nihilistic delusion:

- Theme centers on the nonexistence of self or parts of self, others, or the world
- May have false belief that the world is ending

Delusions of jealousy (infidelity):

- His/her spouse or lover is having an affair

Delusion of guilt/sin/self-accusation:

- Feeling of remorse or guilt of delusional intensity

Delusion of mind being read:

- Other people can know one's thoughts
- Not thought broadcasting, where thoughts are heard aloud

Delusion of reference:

- Insignificant remarks, events, or objects in one's environment have personal meaning or significance
- Special messages from the news anchorperson/television/newspaper

Erotomania:

- One believes that another person, usually someone of higher status, is in love with him/her

Grandiose delusions:

- An individual exaggerates his/her sense of self-importance and is convinced that he/she has special powers, talents, or abilities

Persecutory delusions:

- Theme of being followed, harassed, cheated, poisoned or drugged, conspired against, spied on, attacked, or obstructed in pursuit of goals

Religious delusion:

- Any delusion with religious/spiritual content
- May be combined with others (e.g., grandiose – person chose by God, control, guilt)

Somatic delusion:

- Content pertains to bodily functioning, bodily sensations, or physical appearance
- Body is somehow diseased, abnormal, or changed

Defense Mechanisms

Primitive:

- **Denial** – refusal to accept reality/fact, acting as if a painful event, thought, or feeling did not exist; a/w substance abuse and death
- **Thought blocking** – transient inability to remember
- **Regression** – reversion to an earlier stage of development in the face of unacceptable thoughts or impulses
- **Acting out** – performing an extreme behavior in order to express thoughts or feelings the person feels incapable of otherwise expressing; a/w substance abuse, fighting, gambling
- **Dissociation** – loses track of time and/or person, and instead finds another representation of their self in order to continue in the moment; a/w fugue, depersonalization, amnesia, and DID
- **Compartmentalization** – lesser form of dissociation, wherein parts of oneself are separated from awareness or other parts and behaving as if one had separate sets of values
- **Projection** – misattribution of a person's undesired thoughts, feelings, or impulses onto another person who does not have those thoughts, feelings, or impulses; occurs esp. when the thoughts/feelings are considered unacceptable to have; a/w paranoia
- **Reaction formation** – converting unwanted or dangerous thoughts, feelings, or impulses into their opposites; a/w OCD
- **Splitting** – world is composed of polar opposites (e.g., good vs. evil), a/w borderline PD
- **Somatization** – physical symptoms of psychological reasons (repression expressed through body complaints; anxiety converted into a specific symptom), a/w somatization disorders

Less Primitive:

- **Repression** – unconscious blocking of unacceptable thoughts, feelings, and impulses
- **Displacement** – the redirecting of thoughts, feelings, and impulses directed at one person or object, but taken out upon another person or object; often used when the individual cannot express their feelings toward the individual they are directed at (produces OCD)
- **Isolation of affect** – facts without feeling → la belle indifference → lack of concern about illness
- **Intellectualization** – overemphasis on thinking when confronted with an unacceptable impulse, situation, or behavior without employing any emotions to help mediate and place the thoughts into an emotional context
- **Rationalization** – putting something into a different light or offering a different explanation for one's perceptions or behaviors in the face of a changing reality
- **Undoing** – attempt to take back an unconscious behavior/thought that is unacceptable or hurtful
- **Introjection** – the outside becomes inside (leads directly to guilt, internalization of the superego)
- **Passive-aggressive** – passive nonperformance after promise

Mature (CASH):

- **Compensation** – process of psychologically counterbalancing perceived weakness by emphasizing strength in other arenas; avoids recognition of inability to be strong in all areas
- **Assertiveness** – emphasis of a person's needs or thoughts in a manner that is respectful, direct, and firm; falls between passive and aggressive
- **Sublimation** – channeling unacceptable impulses, thoughts, and emotions into more acceptable ones (vigorous exercise, humor, fantasy, art)
- **Humor** – a pleasant release from anxiety; laughter hides pain

Affective/Mood Disorder

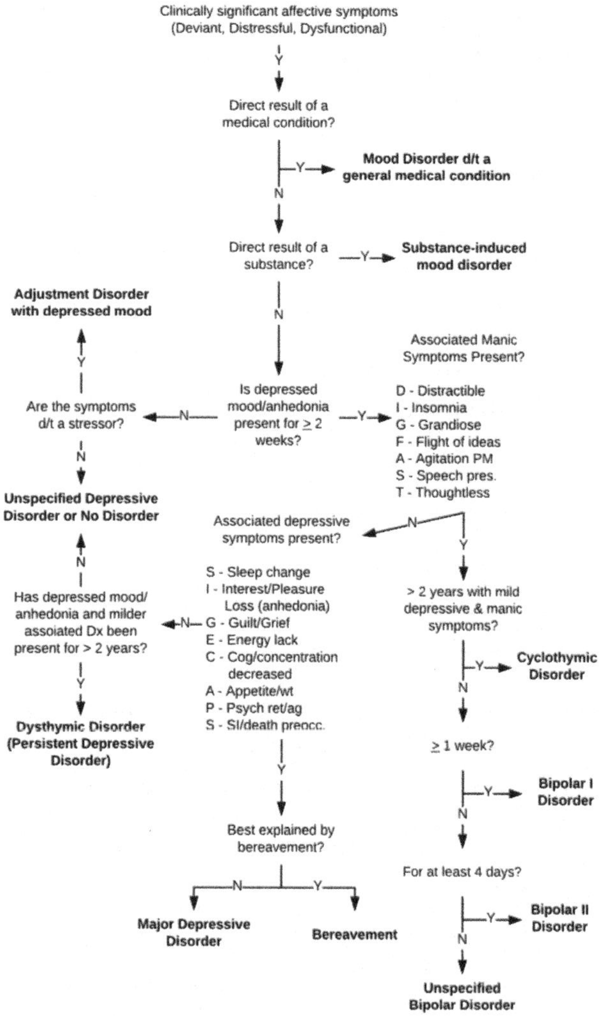

Affective/Mood Disorders

Major Depressive Disorder (MDD)

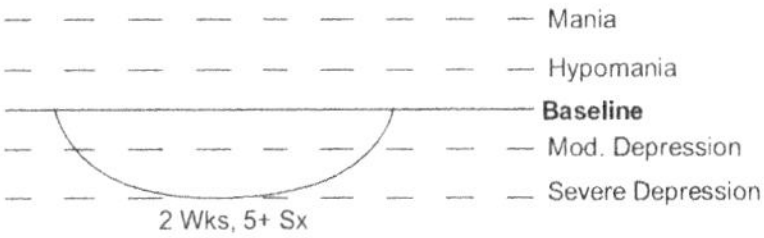

Dysthymic Disorder

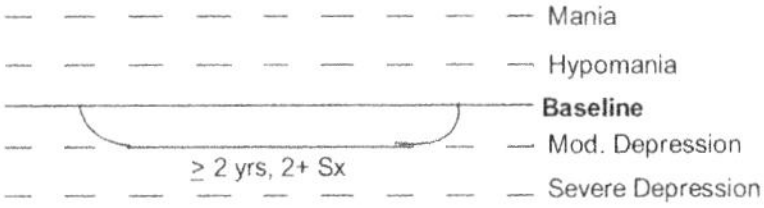

Bipolar I Disorder

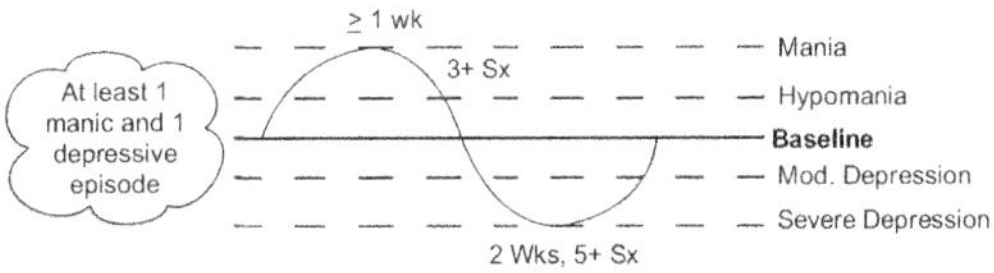

Bipolar II Disorder

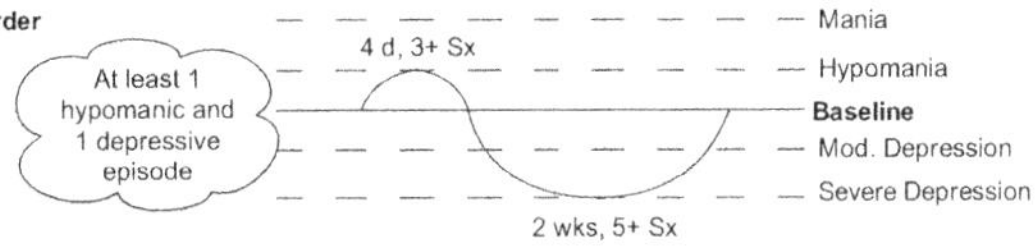

Cyclothymic Disorder

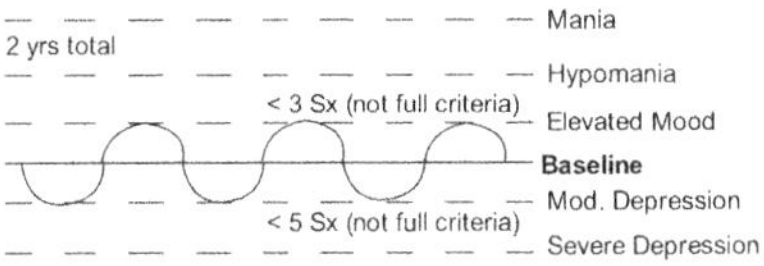

Depression Management

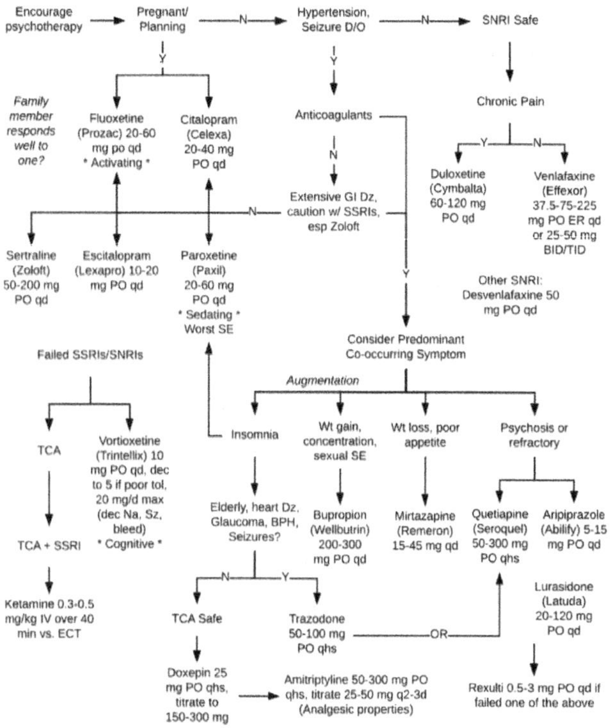

Return after 4-6 week SSRI/SNRI trial (after remission best)

	Ineffective	Partially Effective	Effective
Poor Tolerance	Alternative based on "predominant Sx category" MTHFR → L-methyl folate 7.5 mg PO qd Ferritin → Repl., cofactor	Same class, alternative profile	Alternative based on SE profile
Tolerating Well	Alternative SSRI/SNRI, ?↑dose	↑ dose vs. augment w/ mirtazapine, bupropion, aripiprazole, quetiapine, buspirone	Continue present regimen
W/D: Dizziness/paresthesia most common, 3-4 d after cessation, cross-titrate if high doses; some don't W/D "ever gone without meds?"; relapse highest @ 2 months			

Mania Management

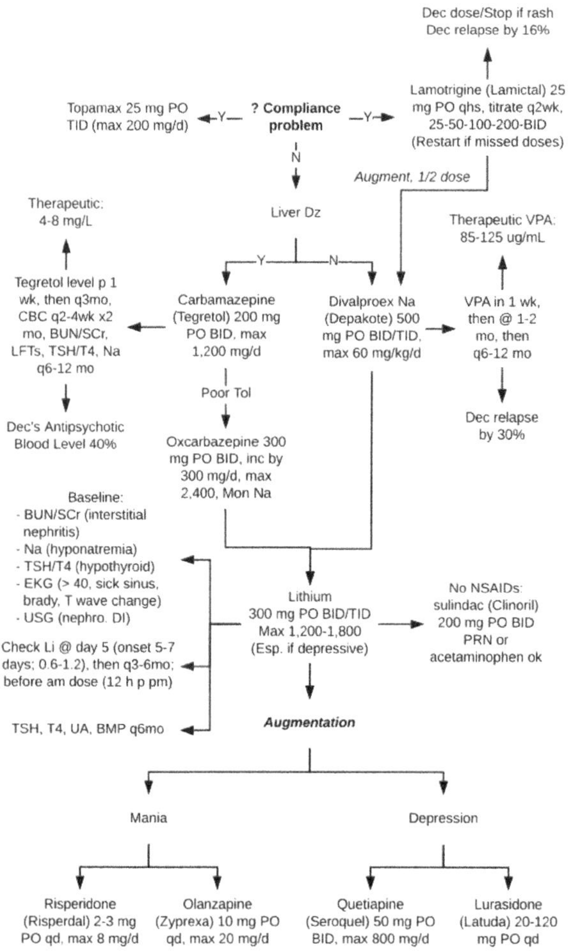

Lithium Toxicity

Amdisen Rating Scale	Lithium Level (mEq/L)	Correlation	Manifestations	Management
0	0.6-1.2	Normal	No S/S	N/A
1	> 1.5	Mild	N/V, tremor, hyperreflexia, agitation, weakness, drowsy	- IV NS - Na polystyrene sulfonate PO - Hemodialysis if severe neuro Sx, renal insufficiency, HD instability, neuro unstable
2	1.5-2.5	Moderate	Stupor, rigidity, hypertonia, hypotension, flat/inv. T's, hyperthermia, ataxia	
3	> 2.5	Severe	Myoclonus, CV collapse, Sz, coma, renal insufficiency	

Psychosis

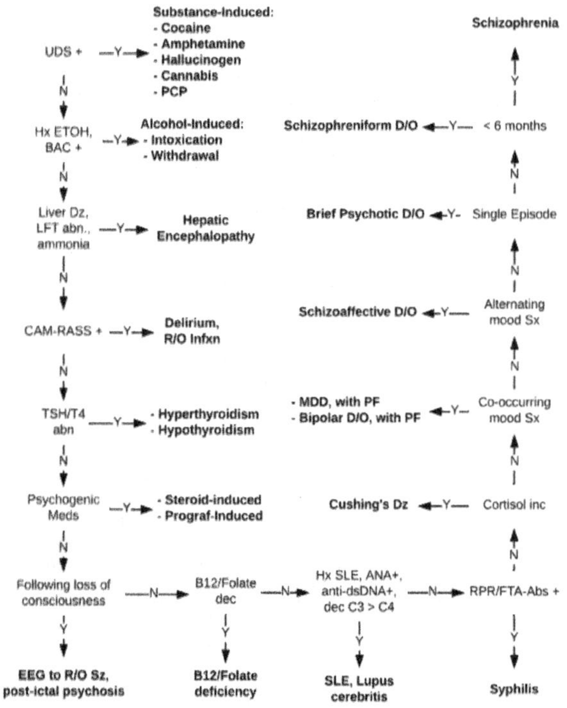

Psychosis Management

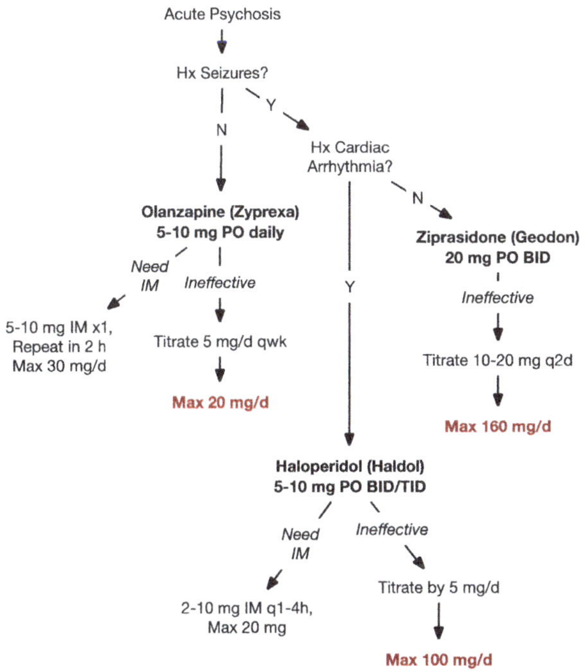

Avoid Ativan if on Zyprexa C/I d/t HoTN

As pt stabilizes, maintain on antipsychotic or switch to antipsychotic based on profile (Step 2).

Modified Psychosis Algorithm (Step 2)

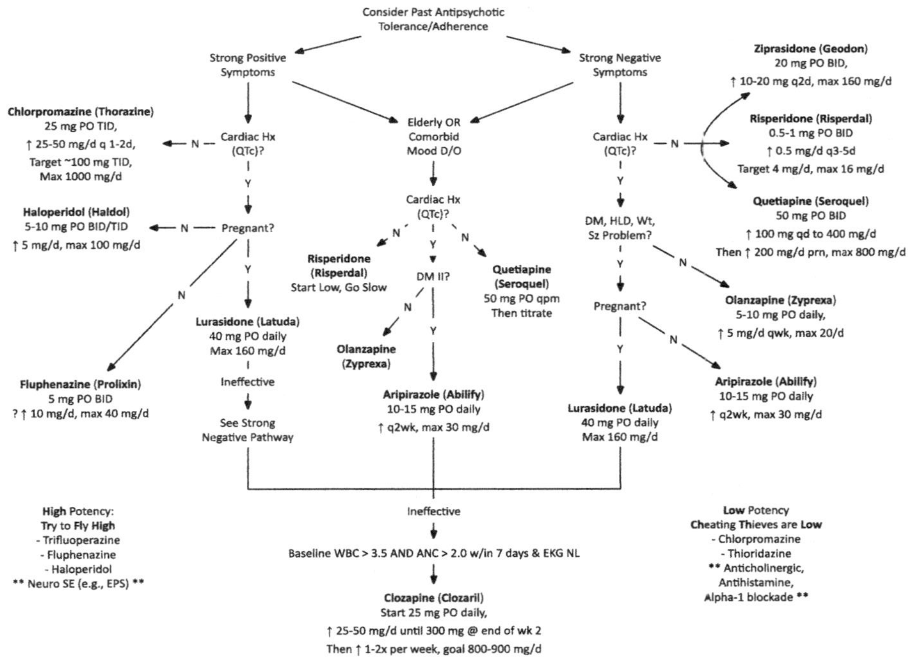

Psychosis Management Algorithm (Step 3)

Consider clozapine (Clozaril), consider early if recurrent suicidality, violence, or comorbid substance abuse with persistent positive symptoms for > 2 years.

Prior to Starting:

- CBC showing WBC $\geq$ 3.5 and ANC $\geq$ 2.0 w/in 7 days
- Baseline EKG

Titrating:

- Doses can be titrated daily in dosage increments of 25-50 mg/day as tolerated to achieve a target dose of 300-450 mg/day at the end of 2 weeks
- After 2 weeks, titrate once/twice weekly
- Titrate cautiously in divided doses to reduce the risk of hypotension, seizure, and sedation
    - May also consider lower am dose with higher pm dose if sedation

Week 1	AM Dose (mg)	PM Dose (mg)	Total Dose (mg)
Day 1	12.5	12.5 ?	12.5-25
Day 2	25	X	25
Day 3	25	25	50
Day 4	25	50	75
Day 5	50	50	100
Day 6	50	75	125
Day 7	50	100	150
Day 8	75	100	175
Day 9	100	100	200
Day 10	100	125	225
Day 11	100	150	250
Day 12	125	150	275
Day 13	150	150	300
Day 14	150	150	300

Monitoring:

- Monitor CBC weekly x 6 months, then q2wk x6 months, then q4wk afterwards
- Annual EKG and echocardiogram

Discontinue if:

- WBC < 3.0 and/or ANC < 1.0

Considerations:

- If 48 hours since last dose, then must restart/re-titrate
- Avoid Tegretol

Clozapine Levels:

- Check 12 h after last dose
- 200-300 ng/mL, medium range, initial target level
- 350-450 ng/mL, high range, no more effective than medium range
- Doubling the dose will double the level

Clozapine + Norclozapine > 1000 ng/mL, no proven benefit, ↑ seizure risk

Extrapyramidal Symptom Management

4 and ADAPT: 4 hours **A**cute **D**ystonia, 4 days **A**kinesia, 4 weeks **A**kathesia, 4 months **P**arkinsonian & **T**D

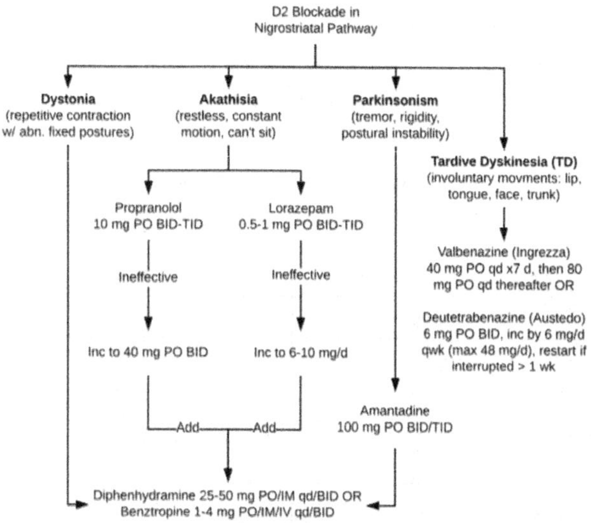

Atropine 1% eye gtts SL, 2 gtt SL qhs

Neuroleptic malignant syndrome (NMS):

- **F** – Fever
- **E** – Encephalopathy
- **V** – Vital sign instability
- **E** – Elevated WBC/CPK
- **R** – Rigidity

Management: Lorazepam 1-4 mg x1; Dantrolene

Common Antipsychotic Side Effects:

- Anticholinergic (can't see, can't pee, can't shit)
- N/V, sedation, OH
- Hormonal (libido, wt gain, amenorrhea)
- EKG changes (prolonged QTI, arrhythmia)
- ↑ risk of seizures

Monitor for HoTN with propranolol and amantadine; sedation & HoTN with lorazepam, CA W/D seizures

Conversion to Decanoate Injections

Haldol Decanoate:

- 10-20 x PO dose
    - 10 mg if elderly, debilitated
    - 20 mg if decompensation, Hx tolerance
- Give no more than 100 mg w/ 1st dose
- F/U with balance in 3-7 days
- Maintenance 10-15 x PO dose q4wk
- Max dose 400 mg/month
- Tmax ~ 1 week

Paliperidone (**Invega Sustenna**):

- 234 mg IM x 1, day one
- 156 mg IM x1, day eight
- 117 mg IM (39-234 mg IM) maintenance
- Administer q 4 wk
- PO not required, but tapering risperidone over 1 wk prevents W/D insomnia

Abilify Maintena:

- 400 mg IM initially
- 300-400 mg IM q 4 weeks for maintenance
- Continue PO dose for 14 days

Fluphenazine (**Prolixin Decanoate**):

- Initially 12.5-25 mg IM
- 12.5 mg IM = 10 mg PO; ~1.25 x PO dose for estimate
- Maintenance, titrate in 12.5 mg increments
- Max 100 mg
- Administer q2 weeks
- Onset 24-48 hours
- ↑ EPS risk w/in 1st 48 hours
    - Prophylaxis w/ Cogentin/Benadryl, D/C if no EPS in 48h
- Steady state in ~2 months
- Continue ½ PO dose

Attention-Deficit Hyperactivity Disorder (ADHD)

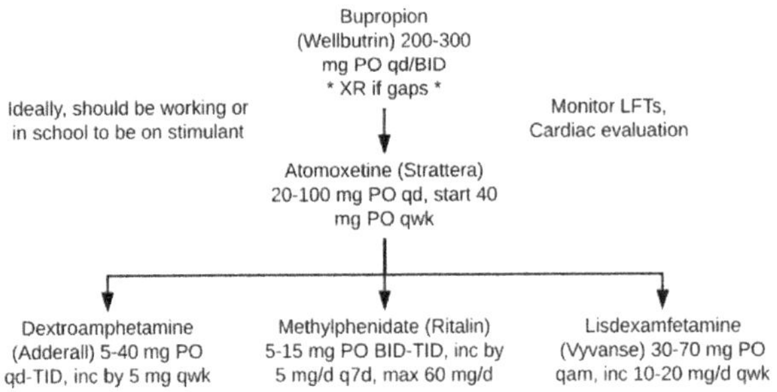

Anxiety

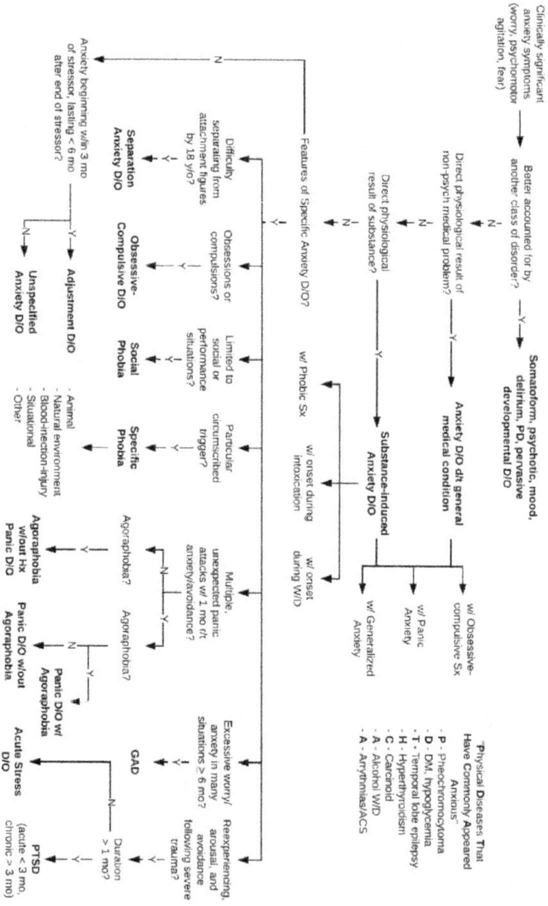

Clinically significant anxiety symptoms (worry, psychomotor agitation, fear)
Better accounted for by another class of disorder?
Somatoform, psychotic, mood, delirium, PD, pervasive developmental D/O
Direct physiological result of non-psych medical problem?
Anxiety D/O d/t general medical condition
w/ Obsessive-compulsive Sx
w/ Panic Anxiety
w/ Generalized Anxiety
"Physical Diseases That Have Commonly Appeared Anxious"
- P - Pheochromocytoma
- D - DM, hypoglycemia
- T - Temporal lobe epilepsy
- H - Hyperthyroidism
- C - Carcinoid
- A - Alcohol W/D
- A - Arrythmias/ACS
Direct physiological result of substance?
Substance-Induced Anxiety D/O
w/ Phobic Sx
w/ onset during intoxication
w/ onset during W/D
Features of Specific Anxiety D/O?
Difficulty separating from attachment figures by 18 y/o?
Separation Anxiety D/O
Obsessions or compulsions?
Obsessive-Compulsive D/O
Limited to social or performance situations?
Social Phobia
Particular circumscribed trigger?
Specific Phobia
- Animal
- Natural environment
- Blood-injection-injury
- Situational
- Other
Multiple, unexpected panic attacks w/ 1 mo f/t anxiety/avoidance?
Agoraphobia?
Agoraphobia w/out Hx Panic D/O
Agoraphobia?
Panic D/O w/ Agoraphobia
Panic D/O w/out Agoraphobia
Excessive worry/ anxiety in many situations ≥ 6 mo?
GAD
Reexperiencing, arousal, and avoidance following severe trauma?
Duration > 1 mo?
Acute Stress D/O
PTSD (acute < 3 mo, chronic > 3 mo)
Anxiety beginning w/in 3 mo of stressor, lasting < 6 mo after end of stressor?
Adjustment D/O
Unspecified Anxiety D/O
Y
N

Anxiety Management

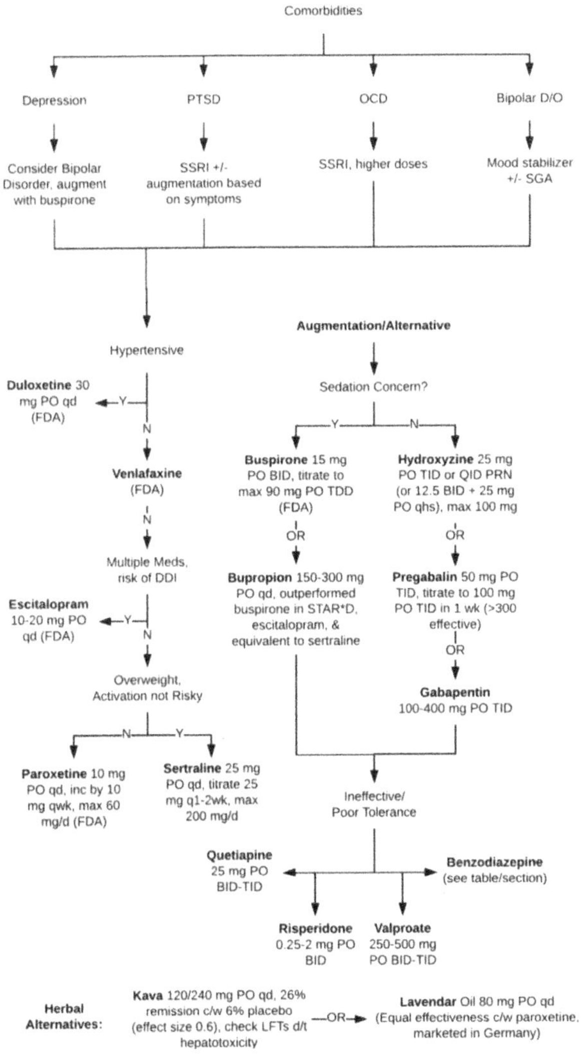

PTSD Management

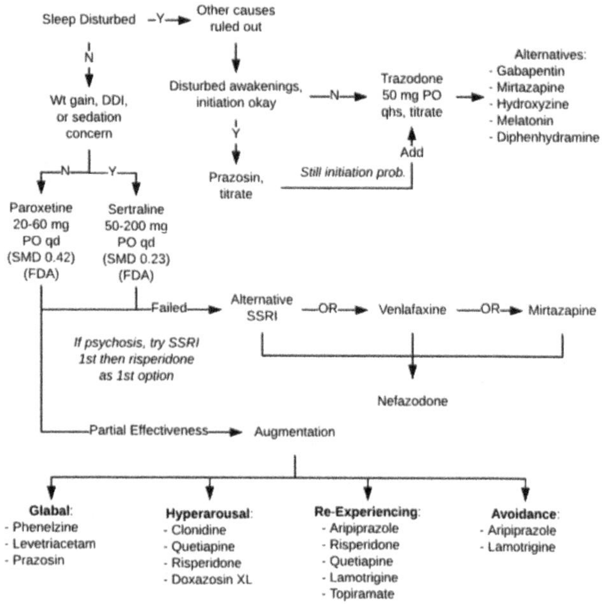

Prazosin Titration

Male		Female	
Bedtime Dose	10-11 am Dose	Bedtime Dose	10-11 am Dose
1 mg PO qhs x 2 2 mg PO qhs x 5 4 mg PO qhs x 7 6 mg PO qhs x 7 10 mg PO qhs x 7 15 mg PO qhs x 7 Max: 25 mg PO qhs	1 mg PO @ 14 days 2 mg PO @ 21-28 days 6 mg PO @ 35+ days	1 mg PO qhs x 3 2 mg PO qhs x 11 4 mg PO qhs x 7 6 mg PO qhs x 7 Max: 10 mg PO qhs	1 mg PO @ 14-21 days 2 mg PO @ 28+ days

Substance Use Disorders (SUDs)

Drug	Intoxication	Withdrawal
Alcohol	Disinhibition, emotional lability, slurred speech, ataxia, aggression, blackouts, hallucinations, memory impairment, impaired judgment, coma	Tremor, tachycardia, HTN, malaise, nausea, seizures, DTs, agitation
Opioids	Euphoria → apathy, CNS depression, constipation, pupillary constriction, and respiratory depression (life-threatening in OD) Naloxone and naltrexone reverse effects, but caution b/c antagonist may clear before opioids	Dysphoria, insomnia, myalgias, fever, lacrimation, diaphoresis, dilated pupils, rhinorrhea, piloerection, N/V, stomach cramps, diarrhea, yawning
Amphet-amines	Psychomotor agitation, impaired judgment, HTN, pupillary dilation, tachycardia, fever, diaphoresis, anxiety, angina, euphoria, prolonged wakefulness/attention, arrhythmias, delusions, seizures, hallucinations BZDs front line; Haloperidol can be given for agitation; symptomatic relief (antiemetics, NSAIDs, etc.)	Post-use crash with anxiety, lethargy, HA, stomach cramps, hunger, fatigue, depression/dysphoria, sleep disturbance, nightmares
Cocaine	Psychomotor agitation, euphoria, impaired judgment, tachycardia, pupillary dilation, HTN, paranoia, hallucination, "cocaine bugs", sudden cardiac death, ischemic changes on EKG with "cocaine chest pain" BZDs front line; Haloperidol for agitation; symptomatic relief (e.g., antihypertensives)	Post-use "crash" with hypersomnolence, depression, malaise, severe craving, angina, suicidality, ↑ appetite, nightmares
PCP	Assaultiveness, belligerence, psychosis, violence, impulsiveness, psychomotor agitation, fever, tachycardia, vertical/horizontal nystagmus, HTN, impaired judgment, ataxia, seizures, delirium BZDs or haloperidol for severe symptoms; otherwise reassurance; acidification of urine/gastric lavage helps eliminate.	Recurrence of intoxication symptoms d/t reabsorption in GIT; sudden onset of severe, random violence.
LSD	Marked anxiety or depression, delusions, visual hallucinations, flashbacks, pupillary dilation, impaired judgment, diaphoresis, tachycardia, HTN, heightened senses (e.g., colors more intense) Supportive counseling/care; traditional antipsychotics & BZDs	None

Cannabis	Euphoria, slowed sense of time, impaired judgment, social withdrawal, ↑ appetite, dry mouth, conjunctival injection, hallucinations, anxiety, paranoia, amotivational syndrome	None
Barbit-urates	Low safety margin; respiratory depression	Anxiety, seizures, delirium, life-threatening cardiovascular collapse
BZDs	Interactions with ETOH, amnesia, ataxia, somnolence, mild respiratory depression (avoid using for insomnia in elderly, paradoxical agitation even in low doses)	Rebound anxiety, seizures, tremor, insomnia, HTN, tachycardia, death
Caffeine	Restlessness, insomnia, diuresis, muscle twitching, arrhythmias, tachycardia, flushed face, psychomotor agitation	Headache, lethargy, depression, weight gain, irritability, craving
Nicotine	Restlessness, insomnia, anxiety, arrhythmias	Irritability, headache, anxiety, weight gain, craving, bradycardia, difficulty concentrating, insomnia

Opioid Cessation Management with naltrexone LAI (Vivitrol)

Opioid free x 7 days, UDS neg → Naltrexone 25 mg PO x1 challenge → 1 hr w/out W/D symptoms → Vivitrol 380 mg IM now & q4wk

Alcohol Withdrawal

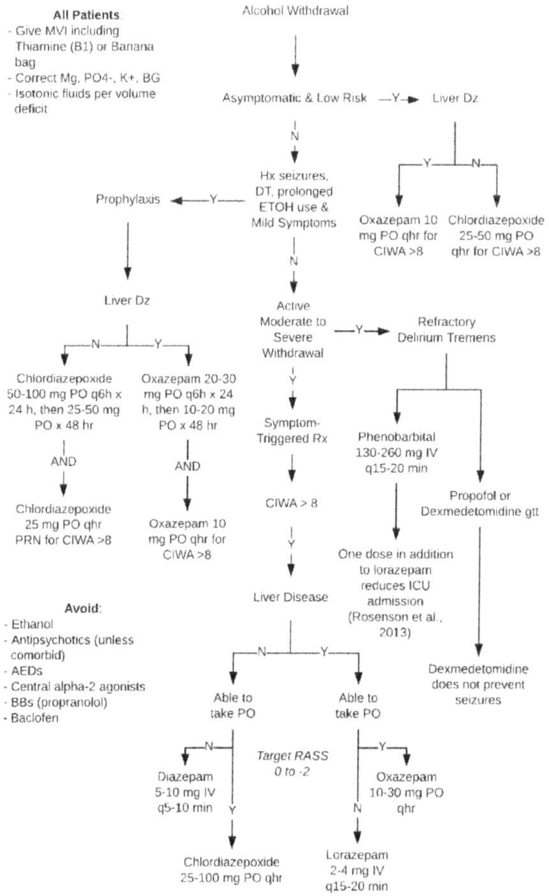

Neurocognitive Disorders

Problem of memory, orientation, judgment, and attention

Variable	Delirium	Dementia
Level of Attention	Impaired (fluctuating)	Usually alert
Onset	Acute	Gradual
Course	Fluctuating from hour to hour "sundowning"	Progressive deterioration
Consciousness	Clouded	Intact
Hallucinations	Present (often visual or tactile)	Occur in approx. 30% pts in advanced Dz
Prognosis	Reversible	Largely irreversible, but 15% cases d/t treatable causes and are reversible
Treatment	- Target underlying cause - Low-dose antipsychotic (Haldol is DOC if hyperactive) - Environmental change - Frequent orientation - Low-stimulus - Glasses, hearing aids, etc.	- Cholinesterase inhibitors - Low-dose antipsychotics (behavioral disturbances) - Environmental changes - Avoid BZDs, exacerbates disinhibition and confusion

Causes of Dementia
"DEMENTIASS"

D – Degenerative Dz (Parkinson, Huntington)

E – Endocrine (thyroid, parathyroid, pituitary, adrenal)

M – Metabolic (alcohol, lytes, vitamin B12 def., glucose, hepatic, renal, Wilson Dz)

E – Exogenous (heavy metals, carbon monoxide, drugs)

N – Neoplasm

T – Trauma (SDH)

I – Infxn (meningitis, encephalitis, endocarditis, syphilis, HIV, prion Dz, Lyme Dz)

A – Affective D/O's (pseudodementia)

SS – Stroke/Structure (vascular dementia, ischemia, vasculitis, normal-pressure hydrocephalus)

Causes of Delirium
"I WATCH DEATH"

I – Infxn

W – Withdrawal

A – Acute metabolic/substance Abuse

T – Trauma

C – CNS pathology

H – Hypoxia

D – Deficiencies

E – Endocrine

A – Acute vascular/MI

T – Toxins/drugs

H – Heavy metals

Delirium

Score	Term	Description
+4	Combative	Overly combative, violent, immediate danger to staff
+3	Very Agitated	Pulls or removes tube(s) or catheter(s); aggressive
+2	Agitated	Frequent non-purposeful movements, fights vent
+1	Restless	Anxious but movements not aggressive, vigorous
0	Alert & Calm	
-1	Drowsy	Not fully alert, but has sustained awakening (eye-opening/eye contact) to voice ($\geq$ 10 sec)
-2	Light Sedation	Briefly awakens with eye contact to voice (< 10 sec)
-3	Moderate Sedation	Movement or eye opening to voice (but no eye contact)
-4	Deep Sedation	No response to voice, but movement or eye opening to physical stimulation
-5	Unarousable	No response to voice or physical stimulation

If RASS above -4 (-3 through +4), then proceed to next step

Acute Onset of Mental Status Changes or a Fluctuating Course

Is there an acute change from mental status baseline? OR
Has the patient's mental status fluctuated during the past 24 hours?

Yes

Inattention

"Squeeze my hand when I say the letter 'A'."
Read to pt: S A V E A H A A R T

> 2 Error

Disorganized Thinking

1. Will a stone float on water?
2. Are there fish in the sea?
3. Does one pound weigh more than two?
4. Can you use a hammer to pound a nail?

Command:
"Hold up this many fingers" (hold up 2 fingers)
"Now do the same thing with the other hand"
(do not demonstrate)
OR "Add one more finger"

OR

Altered LOC

RASS other than zero
(-3, -2, -1, 1, 2, 3, 4)

> 1 Error — Yes

Delirium

Personality Disorders

Weird, Wild, and Worried

Cluster A: Behaviors described as odd or eccentric

- **Weird**: Cluster **A** is **A**ccusatory, **A**loof, & **A**wkward
- Paranoid Personality Disorder (**A**ccusatory)
- Schizoid Personality Disorder (**A**loof)
- Schizotypal Personality Disorder (**A**wkward)

Cluster B: Behaviors described as dramatic, emotional, or erratic

- **Wild**: Cluster **B** is **B**ad, **B**orderline, flam**B**oyant, must be the **B**est
- Antisocial Personality Disorder (**B**ad)
- Borderline Personality Disorder (**B**orderline)
- Histrionic Personality Disorder (flam**B**oyant)
- Narcissistic Personality Disorder (must be the **B**est)

Cluster C: Behaviors described as anxious or fearful

- **Worried**: Cluster **C** is **C**owardly, obsessive-**C**ompulsive, **C**lingy
- Avoidant Personality Disorder (**C**owardly)
- Obsessive-Compulsive Personality Disorder (obsessive-**C**ompulsive)
- Dependent Personality Disorder (**C**lingy)

Histrionic

- **P** – Provocative or seductive Bx
- **R** – Relationships considered more intimate than they actually are
- **A** – Attention (need to be center of)
- **I** – Influenced easily
- **S** – Style of speech (impressionistic, lacking detail)
- **E** – Emotions (rapidly shifting, shallow)
- **M** – Make up (physical appearance used to draw attention to self)
- **E** – Emotions exaggerated

Avoidant

- **C** – Criticism or rejection preoccupies thoughts in social situations
- **R** – Restraint in relationships d/t fear of shame
- **I** – Inhibited in new relationships
- **N** – Needs to be sure of being liked before engaging socially
- **G** – Gets around occupational activities w/ need for interpersonal contact
- **E** – Embarrassment prevents new activity or taking risks
- **S** – Self viewed as unappealing or inferior

Dependent

- **R** – Reassurance required
- **E** – Expressing disagreement difficult
- **L** – Life responsibilities assumed by others
- **I** – Initiating projects difficult
- **A** – Alone (feels helpless and uncomfortable when alone)
- **N** – Nurturance (goes to excessive lengths to obtain)
- **C** – Companionship sought urgently when a relationship ends
- **E** – Exaggerated fears of being left to care for self

Paranoid

- **S** – Spousal infidelity suspected
- **U** – Unforgiving (bears grudges)
- **S** – Suspicious
- **P** – Perceives attacks (and reacts quickly)
- **E** – Enemy or friend? (suspects associates and friends)
- **C** – Confiding in others is feared
- **T** – Threats perceived in benign events

Schizoid

- **D** – Detached or flattened affect
- **I** – Indifferent to criticism or praise
- **S** – Sexual experiences of little interest
- **T** – Tasks done solitarily
- **A** – Absence of close friends
- **N** – Neither desires nor enjoys close relationships
- **T** – Takes pleasure in few activities

Narcissistic

- **G** – Grandiose
- **R** – Requires attention
- **A** – Arrogant
- **N** – Needs to be special
- **D** – Dreams of success and power
- **I** – Interpersonally exploitative
- **O** – Others (unable to recognize feelings/needs)
- **S** – Sense of entitlement
- **E** – Envious

Schizotypal

- **M** – Magical thinking
- **E** – Experiences unusual perceptions
- **P** – Paranoid ideation
- **E** – Eccentric Bx or appearance
- **C** – Constricted/inappropriate affect
- **U** – Unusual thinking or speech
- **L** – Lacks close friends
- **I** – Ideas of reference
- **A** – Anxiety in social situations
- **R** – Rule out psychotic or pervasive developmental D/O's

Antisocial

- **C** – Cannot conform to law
- **O** – Obligations ignored
- **R** – Reckless disregard for safety
- **R** – Remorseless
- **U** – Underhanded (deceitful)
- **P** – Planning insufficient (impulsive)
- **T** – Temper (irritable and aggressive)

Obsessive-Compulsive

- **S** – Stubborn
- **C** – Cannot discard worthless objects
- **R** – Rule obsessed
- **I** – Inflexibility
- **M** – Miserly
- **P** – Perfectionistic
- **E** – Excludes leisure d/t devotion to work
- **R** – Reluctant to delegate to others

Borderline

- **I** – Impulsive
- **M** – Moodiness
- **P** – Paranoia or dissociation under stress
- **U** – Unstable self-image
- **L** – Labile intense relationships
- **S** – Suicidal gestures
- **I** – Inappropriate anger
- **V** – Vulnerability to abandonment
- **E** – Emptiness (feeling of)

- **D** – Disturbance of identity
- **E** – Emotionally labile
- **S** – Suicidal Bx
- **P** – Paranoia or dissociation
- **A** – Abandonment (fear of)
- **I** – Impulsive
- **R** – Relationships unstable
- **E** – Emptiness (feeling of)
- **R** – Rage (inappropriate)

Somatoform and Feigning Disorders

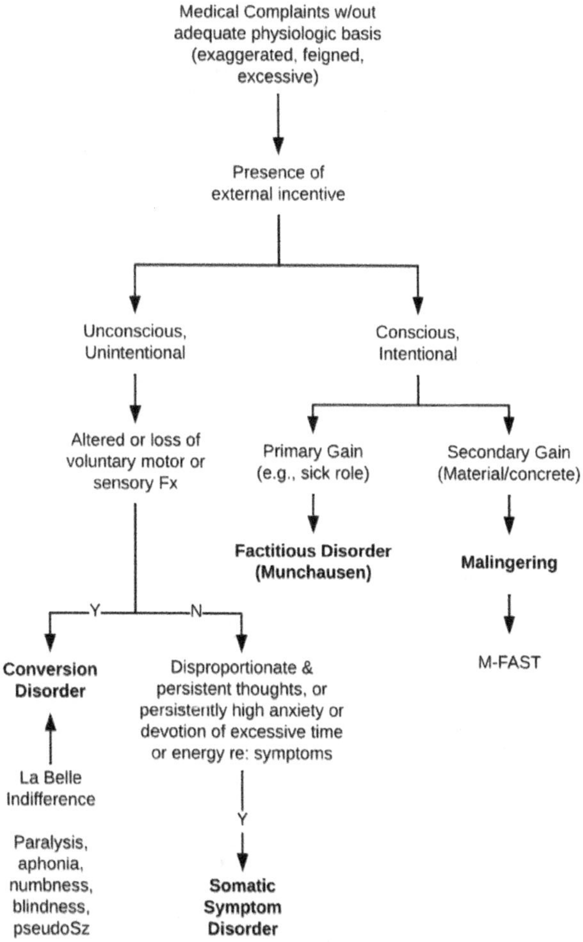

Critical Care & Trauma

Trauma

A – Airway

- Talking → airway patent → frequent reassessment
- Unable to talk → eval for facial fracture/tracheal/laryngeal injury/other obstruction
    - If obstruction not reversible w/ chin lift jaw thrust or GCS < 8, then intubate w/ C-spine immobilization
- Severe facial/neck trauma be prepared for Sx airway

B – Breathing/Ventilation

- Evaluate chest wall excursion/bilat breath sounds/chest wall (flail chest, crepitance, open chest wound, tracheal injury)
- Identify/repair injuries that impair ventilation
- Tension PTX (needle decompression/finger or tube thoracostomy)
- Flail chest w/ pulmonary contusion, massive hemothorax → tube thoracostomy
    - If > 1,500 mL blood out or > 200 mL/h or HD unstable, then OR

C – Circulation

- Hypotension, AMS, confusion, mottled skin, thready/diminished pulse
    - Hemorrhage/hypovolemia until proven o/w
    - Place multiple large-bore IVs
    - Control external hemorrhage
    - Resuscitate w/ 2L NS
    - Transfuse PRBCs (males O+, females O-)
    - Consider massive x-fusion protocol (1PRBC:1FFP:1Plt) if persistent transfusion requirements
    - Permissive HoTN (SBP 70 – 100 mmHg) improves mortality

D – Disability

- Rapid neuro assessment
- AVPU
    - Alert
    - Responds to Verbal stimuli
    - Responds to Pain
    - Unresponsive
- GCS

E – Environmental/Exposure

- Remove clothes
- Avoid hypothermia (massive x-fusions/environmental exposures)
    - Can lead to coagulopathies
    - Use warmed blankets/IVF

Hypotension

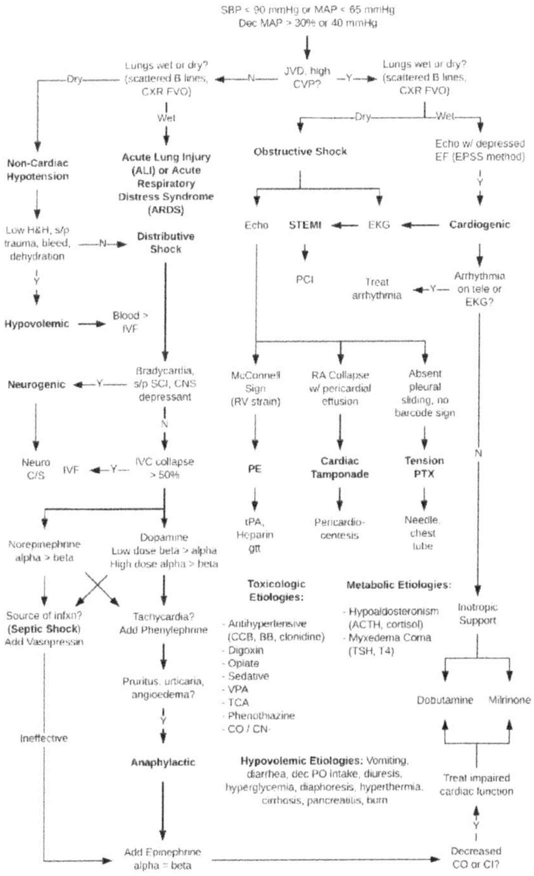

Hemodynamics

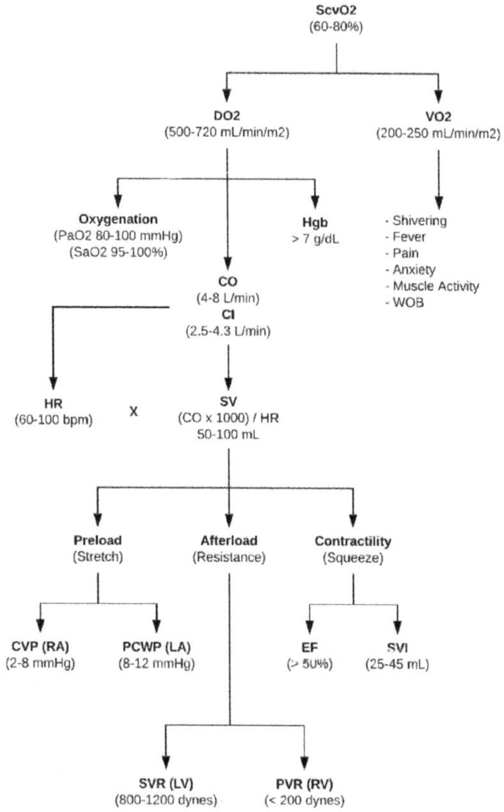

$ScvO_2$

Effectiveness of peripheral O2 delivery

$ScvO_2 < 60\%$	$ScvO_2 > 80\%$
- ↓O_2 supply (↓CO, ↓FiO2, anemia) - ↑ O_2 demand (fever, shivering, ↑ WOB)	- ↑O_2 Supply (FiO_2 > Need) - ↓O_2 demand (hypothermia) - ↓effective O_2 delivery & uptake by cells (sepsis, shift of OHDC to left)

DO_2

"What's delivered to the Toes"

CI x (Hgb x 1.34) x SaO_2 x 10

$DO_2 < 500$ mL/min/m^2	$DO_2 > 720$ mL/min/m^2
- Hemoglobinopathy/anemia - Poor oxygenation, low FiO_2 - Low cardiac output states	- Over-oxygenated, high FiO_2 - High cardiac output states

VO_2

"What's returned", O2 consumed via aerobic metabolism, estimates demand

$VO_2 < 200$ mL/min/m^2	$VO_2 > 250$ mL/min/m^2
- Shivering - Fever - Pain - Anxiety - Muscle activity - Work of breathing (WOB)	- ↓ cellular utilization

CO & CI

Blood Ejected from one ventricle in one minute

CO < 4, CI < 2.5	CO > 8, CI > 4.3
- Inadequate LV Filling - Dysrhythmia - Hypovolemia - Cardiac Tamponade - Mitral/Tricuspid Stenosis - Pericarditis - Restrictive Cardiomyopathy - Inadequate LV Ejection - MI w/ LV failure - Mitral insufficiency - ↑ afterload (HTN, aortic stenosis) - Metabolic disorders - Negative inotropic drugs - Myocardial Dz (myocarditis, cardiomyopathies) - Cardiogenic shock if CI < 2.2 L/min	- Hyperdynamic States - Sepsis - Anemia - Pregnancy - Hyperthyroidism - Thyroid Storm

SV & SVI

Amount of blood ejected from ventricle w/ each heartbeat

SV < 50, SVI < 25	SV > 100, SVI > 45
See factors that increase and decrease variables of preload, afterload, and contractility.	

CVP

Amount of blood returning to the right heart (right atrium)

CVP < 2 mmHg	CVP > 8 mmHg
- Deep inhalation - ↓ vascular tone (distributive shock) - Hypovolemia - Intravascular volume depletion	- Forced exhalation - Tension PTX - Pulmonary HTN - Pleural effusion - Mechanical ventilation (PEEP) - Mitral valve Dz - Hypervolemia - Cardiac tamponade - Right ventricular failure

PCWP

Amount of blood returning to the left heart (left atrium)

PCWP < 8 mmHg	PCWP > 12 mmHg

- Hypovolemia	- Left heart dysfunction
	  - Mitral stenosis/insufficiency
	  - LV failure
	  - ↓ LV compliance)
	- Intravascular volume overload
	- Cardiac tamponade/effusion

SVR

Left Ventricular Afterload, ↓ pulse pressure → ↑ SVR

SVR < 800 dynes/sec/cm^{-5}	SVR < 1,200 dynes/sec/cm^{-5}

- Vasodilation
  - Sepsis
  - Anaphylaxis
  - Vasodilators
  - Hyperthermia
  - End-stage cirrhosis
- ↑ Intra-Thoracic Pressure (PEEP)
- ↑ blood viscosity (severe anemia)
	- Vasoconstriction
	  - Hypertension
	  - Vasopressors
	  - Late sepsis
	  - Hypothermia
	  - Compensation for hypovolemia or low CO
	  - Excessive sympathetic ANS response

PVR

Right Ventricular Afterload, hypoxemia & acidosis → ↑ PVR

PVR > 200	N/A
- Large PE - Pulmonary edema - Hypercapnia - Hypoxemia - Pulmonary HTN	N/A

Contractility (SVI, LVSWI, RVSWI)

Velocity & extent of myocardial fiber shortening

↓ Contractility	↑ Contractility
- Excessive preload or afterload - Negative inotropes - Myocardial damage - Ischemia - Cardiomyopathy - Changes in ionic environment (hypoxemia, acidosis, lyte issues)	- Positive Inotropes - Stimulation of sympathetic ANS - Hyperdynamic states - Hyperthyroidism - Adrenal medulla tumor

Vasopressors

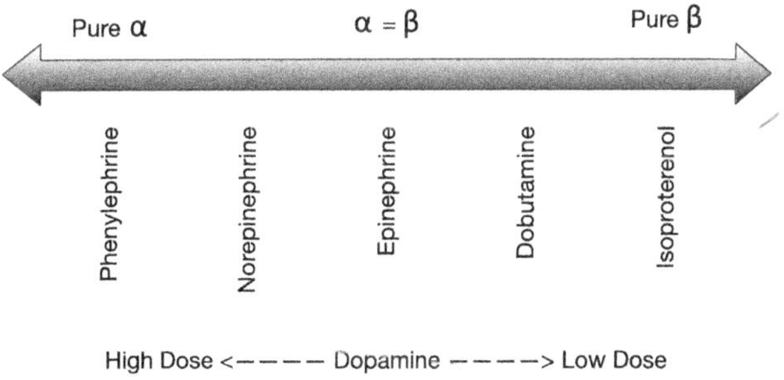

Hemodynamic Variable Management

BP	PCWP	CO	SVR	Plan
↓	↓	↓	↓	Volume
NL	↑	NL	↑	Venodilator/Diuretic
↓	↑	↓	↑	Inotrope
↑	↑	↓	↑	Vasodilator
↓/↑	↑	↓	↑	Inotrope, Vasodilator, IABP
↓	NL	NL/↑	↓	Alpha Agent

Contractility	
↑	↓
- Sympathomimetics (DA, Epi, NE) - PDE-I (milrinone) - Beta agonists (dobutamine) - Dig (not for acute!)	- Beta blockers - Calcium channel blockers - Primarily done to reduce cardiac work and ↓ myocardial O2 demand or reduce outflow obstruction in HCM

Afterload	
↑ (Vasopressors)	↓ (Vasodilators)
- Sympathomimetics - Vasopressin - Ensure adequate preload - 3-5 min response time between dose titrations	- Direct arterial vasodilators (nitroprusside, hydralazine) - ACE-I - CCBs - IABP - RV afterload (O2, pulmonary Vasodilators)

Sepsis

SIRS	> 2 of the following: - Temp > 100.4 or < 96.8 - WBC > 12k OR < 4k - Heart Rate > 90 bpm - Bandemia > 10% - RR > 20, PaCO2 < 32 or on ventilator
SEPSIS	2+ SIRS Criteria + Known or Suspected Infection
SEVERE SEPSIS	Sepsis + Acute Organ Dysfunction (SOFA Criteria) evidenced by: - Resp Failure (Vent, BiPAP) - SpO2 < 90% - Lactic Acid (LA) > 2 - Creatinine > 1.2, acutely - PTT > 60 sec - INR > 1.5 (not on warfarin) - Platelets < 150,000 - T. bilirubin > 1.2 - SBP < 90 or 40 mmHg ↓ from baseline - MAP < 65 - AMS without neuro cause
SEPTIC SHOCK	Severe Sepsis + Hypotension (MAP < 65 mmHg) post 30 mL/kg fluid bolus **OR** Lactic Acid ≥ 4

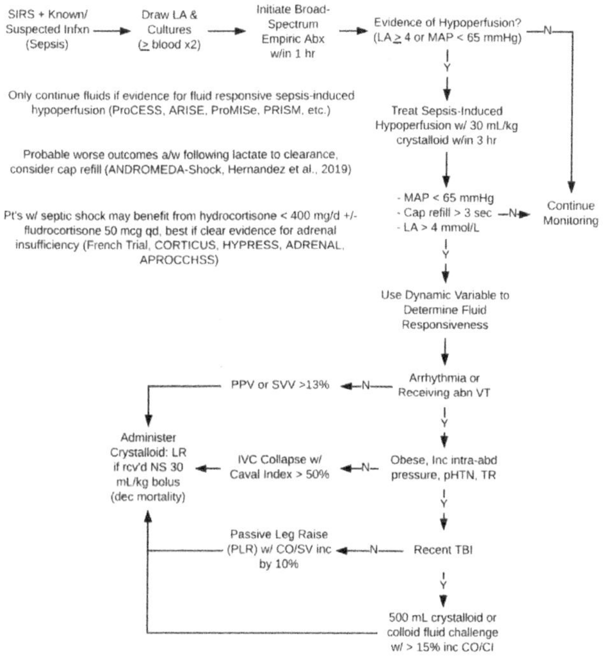

Point of Care Ultrasound (POCUS)

Parasternal Long Axis (PLAX)

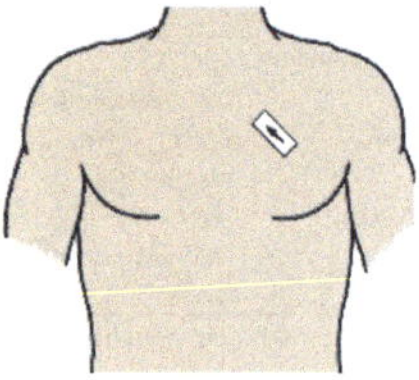

3rd or 4th intercostal space, probe marker to right shoulder

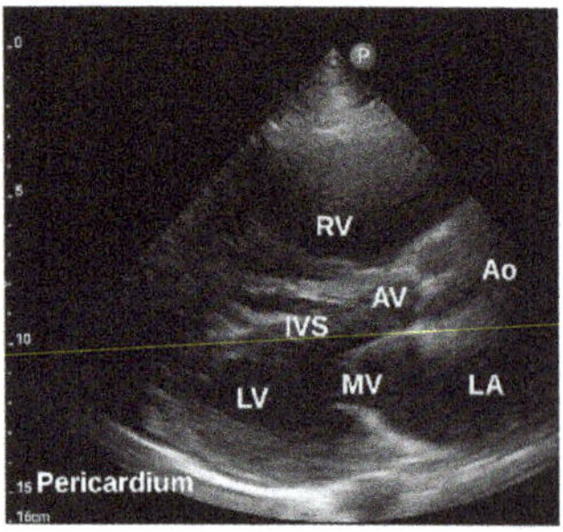

Ao, Aortic Outflow; AV, Aortic Valve; IVS, Intraventricular Septum; LA, Left Atrium; LV, Left Ventricle; MV, Mitral Valve; RV, Right Ventricle

Pericardial effusion: Fluid outside pericardium (deep hyperechoic line)

End-Point Septal Separation (EPSS)

Change to M Mode

Drop line over tip of anterior leaflet

Overestimation:
- Atrial fibrillation
- Septal hypertrophy
- Wall motion abnormalities

Underestimation:
- Mitral stenosis
- Severe mitral regurgitation
- Moderate to severe aortic regurg

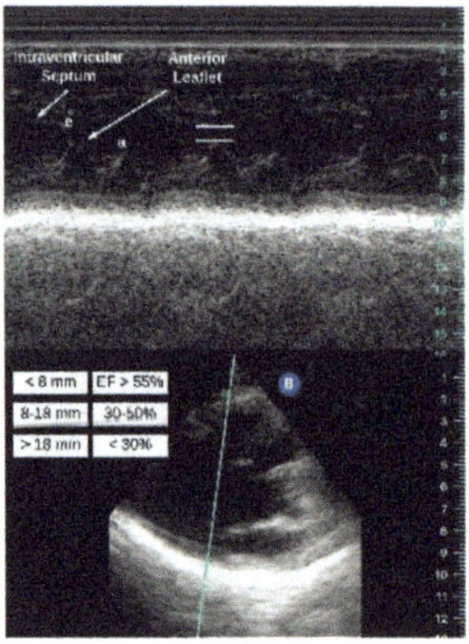

Distance	Ejection Fraction
< 8 mm	> 55%
8 – 18 mm	30 – 50%
> 18 mm	< 30%

IVC Evaluation

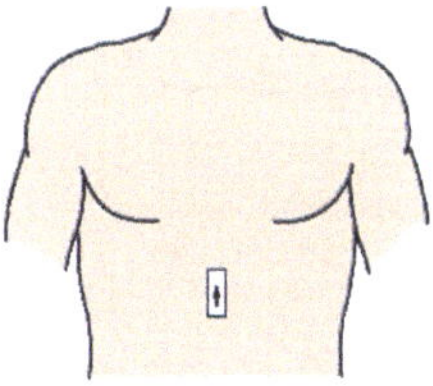

Probe below xyphoid, marker toward head. If collapse > 50% w/ respiration, then volume down.

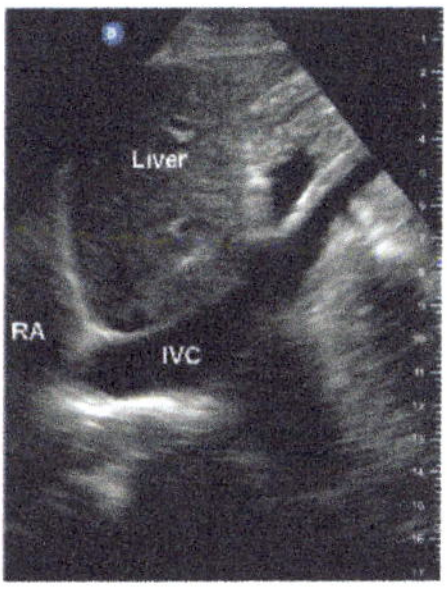

Pulmonary US

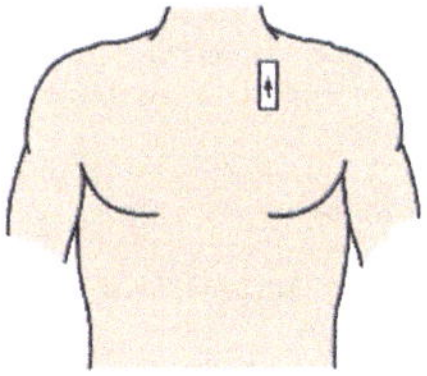

Move probe to each intercostal space.

Should see pleural line superficially ("crawling ants") – lack of "crawling ants" correlates with pneumothorax

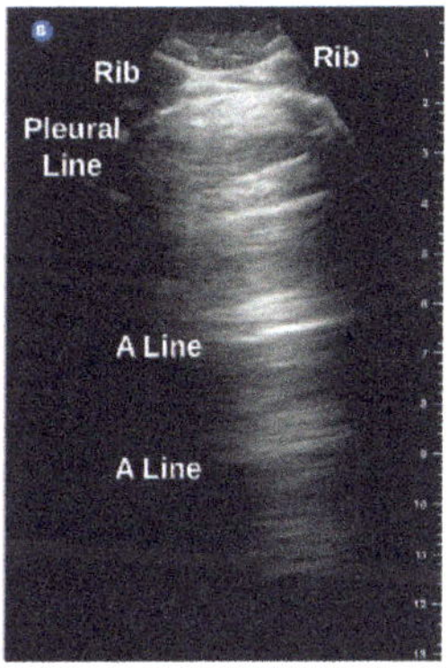

Should see repeating A lines (horizontal lines). "Comet tails" or B lines (vertical lines), correlate with Kerley B lines and indicate fluid (blood, pus, edema) or NL V/Q mismatch (lower lobes). Will never see B lines with A lines.

Abbreviations

5-HIAA: 5-Hydroxyindoleacetic acid
A1c: Hemoglobin A1c
AAA: Abdominal aortic aneurysm
AAT: Alpha-1 antitrypsin
Ab(s): Antibody(ies)
ABC: Airway, breathing, circulation
ABG: Arterial blood gas
ABI: Ankle-brachial index
Abn: Abnormal
ABPA: Allergic bronchopulmonary aspergillosis
Abx: Antibiotic
ACE: Angiotensin converting enzyme
ACE-I: Angiotensin converting enzyme inhibitor
ACS: Acute coronary syndrome
ACTH: Adrenocorticotrophic hormone
ADA: Adenosine deaminase
ADHF: Acute decompensated heart failure
ADL: Activities of daily living
AEC: Absolute eosinophil count
AECOPD: Acute exacerbation of COPD
AED: Antiepileptic drug
AF: Atrial fibrillation
AFB: Acid-fast bacillus
AFL: Atrial flutter
AFP: Alpha fetoprotein
AGEP: Acute generalized exanthematous pustulosis
AGN: Acute glomerulonephritis
AH: Auditory hallucination
AI: Autoimmune
AICD: Automatic implantable cardioverter defibrillator
AIDS: Acquired immunodeficiency syndrome
AIN: Acute Interstitial nephritis
AKI: Acute kidney injury
ALP: Alkaline phosphatase
ALS: Amyotrophic lateral sclerosis
ALT: Alanine aminotransferase
AMS: Altered mental status
ANA: Antinuclear antibody
ANCA: Anti-neutrophil cytoplasmic antibody
ANS: Autonomic nervous system
Anti-CCP: Anti-cyclic citrullinated peptide
Anti-GBM: Anti-glomerular basement membrane
AOM: Acute otitis media
ARDS: Acute respiratory distress syndrome
ASA: Aspirin
ASCVD: Atherosclerotic cardiovascular disease
Asp: Aspiration
AST: Aspartate aminotransferase
ATN: Acute tubular necrosis
AVM: Arteriovenous malformation
A/W: Associated with
BAC: Bronchioloalveolar carcinoma
BAL: Bronchoalveolar lavage
BB: Beta blocker
BCG: Bacille Calmette guerin
BCr: Baseline creatinine
BCx: Blood culture
BG: Blood glucose
BiPAP: Bilevel positive airway pressure
BMBx: Bone marrow biopsy
BMP: Basic metabolic panel
BNP: Brain natriuretic peptide
BOOP: Bronchiolitis obliterans organizing pneumonia
BP: Blood pressure
BPPV: Benign paroxysmal positional vertigo
BR: Bedrest
BRBPR: Bedrest with bathroom privileges
BT: Bleeding time
BUN: Blood urea nitrogen
BVM: Bag-valve-mask
Bx: Behavior/Biopsy
BZD: Benzodiazepine
CA: Cancer
CABG: Coronary artery bypass graft
CAD: Coronary artery disease
CAM-RASS: Confusion assessment method Richmond agitation-sedation scale
CaO2: Arterial oxygen content
CAP: Community-acquired pneumonia
CBC: Complete blood count
CCB: Calcium channel blocker
CEA: Carcinoembryonic antigen
CF: Cystic fibrosis
CFTR: Cystic fibrosis transmembrane conductance regulator
CHD: Congenital heart disease
CI: Cardiac index
CK: Creatinine kinase
CKD: Chronic kidney disease
CM: Case manager
CMP: Complete metabolic panel
CMRI: Cardiac magnetic resonance imaging
CMV: Cytomegalovirus
CN: Cranial nerve
CNS: Central nervous system

CO: Cardiac output
CO2: Carbon dioxide
COP: Cryptogenic organizing pneumonia
COPD: Chronic obstructive pulmonary disease
CP: Chest pain
CPAP: Continuous positive airway pressure
CPPD: Calcium pyrophosphate dihydrate (crystal deposition disease)
CrCl: Creatinine clearance
CRH: Corticotropin releasing hormone
CRP: C-reactive protein
C/S: Consult
CSF: Cerebrospinal fluid
CT: Computed tomography
CTA: Computed tomography angiography
CTEPH: Chronic thromboembolic pulmonary hypertension
CTD: Connective tissue disease
CT Dz: Connective tissue disease
CV: Cardiovascular
CVA: Cerebrovascular accident
CVO2: Mixed venous oxygen content
CVP: Central venous pressure
CW: Chest wall
Cx: Culture
CXR: Chest x-ray
CYP: Cytochrome P450
DAT: Direct antiglobulin test
D/C: Discontinue/Discharge
DCM: Dilated cardiomyopathy
DDx: Differential diagnosis
DHEA: Dehydroepiandrosterone
DI: Diabetes insipidus
DIC: Disseminated intravascular coagulation
DIP: Distal interphalangeal joint
DKA: Diabetic ketoacidosis
DLCO: Diffusion capacity of the lungs for carbon monoxide
DM: Diabetes mellitus
DMARD: Disease-modifying antirheumatic drug
D/O: Disorder
DO2: Oxygen delivery
DOC: Drug of choice
DOE: Dyspnea on exertion
DRESS: Drug reaction with eosinophilia and systemic symptoms
D/T: Due to
DTR: Deep tendon reflexes
DVT: Deep vein thrombosis
DWT: Daily weight
DysFx: Dysfunction
Dx: Diagnosis
Dz: Disease
EBV: Epstein-Barr virus
ED: Erectile dysfunction
EEG: Electroencephalogram
EF: Ejection fraction
EGD: Esophagogastroduodenoscopy
EGPA: Eosinophilic granulomatosis with polyangiitis
EKG: Electrocardiogram
EMG: Electromyelogram
ELISA: Enzyme-linked immunoassay
Eos: Eosinophils
EP: Electrophysiology
EPA: Electrophysiological ablation
EPO: Erythropoietin
EPSS: End-point septal separation
ERCP: Endoscopic retrograde cholangiopancreatography
ESR: Erythrocyte sedimentation rate
ESRD: End-stage renal disease
ETOH: Alcohol
ETT: Endotracheal tube
EUS: Endoscopic ultrasound
FAST: Focused assessment with sonography in trauma
FBG: Fasting blood glucose
F/C: Fever/chills
F/C/R: Fever/chills/rigidity
FDP: Fibrin degradation products
FFP: Fresh frozen plasma
FGA: First generation antipsychotic
FH: Family history
FiO2: Fraction of inspired oxygen
FNA: Fine needle aspiration
FSH: Follicle-stimulating hormone
FTA-ABS: Fluorescent treponemal antibody absorbed
F/U: Follow-up
FVD: Fluid volume deficit
FVO: Fluid volume overload
Fx: Fracture, Function
G-: Gram negative
G+: Gram positive
G6PD: Glucose-6-phosphate dehydrogenase deficiency
GB: Gallbladder
GBS: Guillain-Barre syndrome
GERD: Gastroesophageal reflux disease
GFR: Glomerular filtration rate
GGO: Ground-glass opacities
GI: Gastrointestinal
GN/CL: Gonorrhea/chlamydia
GS: Gram stain
H&H: Hemoglobin & Hematocrit
HA: Headache
HAART: Highly active antiretroviral therapy
HCC: Hepatocellular carcinoma
hCG: Human chorionic gonadotropin
HCTZ: Hydrochlorothiazide

HD: Hemodialysis/Hemodynamic
HDL: High-density lipoprotein
HF: Heart failure
HFNC: High-flow nasal cannula
HFpEF: Heart failure with preserved ejection fraction
HFrEF: Heart failure with reduced ejection fraction
HIDA: Hepatobiliary iminodiacetic acid
HIT: Heparin-induced thrombocytopenia
HIV: Human immunodeficiency virus
HL: Hodgkin's lymphoma
HLD: Hyperlipidemia
HOB: Head of bed
HoTN: Hypotension
HPO: Hypothalamus pituitary ovarian axis
HR: Heart rate
HRCT: High resolution computerized tomography
HSCT: Hematopoietic stem cell transplant
HSP: Hypersensitivity pneumonitis
HSV: Herpes simplex virus
HTN: Hypertension
HUS: Hemolytic uremic syndrome
Hx: History
IBD: Inflammatory bowel disease
IBS: Irritable bowel syndrome
ICD: Implantable cardioverter-defibrillator
ICH: Intracerebral hemorrhage
ICS: Incentive spirometry
IDA: Iron-deficiency anemia
IE: Infective endocarditis
IFNα: Interferon alpha
IICP: Increased intracranial pressure
IIOP: Increased intraocular pressure
IJ: Internal jugular
ILD: Interstitial lung disease
Infxn: Infection
INH: Isoniazid, inhale(r)
INR: International normalized ratio
I/O: Intake and output
IPF: Idiopathic pulmonary fibrosis
ITP: Idiopathic/immune thrombocytopenia purpura
IUD: Intrauterine device
IUP: Intrauterine pregnancy
IVC: Inferior vena cava
IVDU: Intravenous drug use
IVF: Intravenous fluid
IVIG: Intravenous immunoglobulin
JVD: Jugular venous distention
JVP: Jugular venous pressure
KUB: Kidney ureter bladder
LABA: Long-acting beta agonist
LAM: Lymphangioleiomyomatosis
LAMA: Long-acting muscarinic antagonist
LAD: Lymphadenopathy
LBO: Large bowel obstruction
LBP: Low back pain
LDH: Lactate dehydrogenase
LDL: Low-density lipoprotein
LFTs: Liver function tests
LGIB: Low gastrointestinal bleed
LH: Luteinizing hormone
LHF: Left heart failure
Li: Lithium
LIS: Low intermittent suction
LP: Lumbar puncture
LR: Lactated ringers
LT: Long-term
LVEF: Left ventricular ejection fraction
LVSWI: Left ventricular stroke work index
Lytes: Electrolytes
MAC: Mycobacterium avium complex
MAP: Mean arterial pressure
MCV: Mean corpuscular volume
MDI: Metered-dose inhaler
MDR: Multi-drug resistant
MDS: Myelodysplastic syndrome
MEN: Multiple endocrine neoplasia
MG: Myasthenia gravis
MHA-TP: Microhemagglutination assay
MI: Myocardial infarction
MM: Multiple myeloma
MOI: Mechanism of injury
MPGN: Membranoproliferative glomerulonephritis
MRI: Magnetic resonance imaging
MRSA: Methicillin-resistant staphylococcus aureus
MS: Multiple sclerosis
MTHFR: Methylenetetrahydrofolate reductase
MTX: Methotrexate
MV: Minute ventilation, mechanical ventilation
NAAT: Nucleic acid amplification test
NAC: Not a candidate
NHL: Non-Hodgkin's lymphoma
NM: Neuromuscular
NMB: Neuromuscular blocker
NMS: Neuroleptic malignant syndrome
NPO: Nothing per oral
NRB: Non-rebreather
NS: Normal saline
NSAID: Non-steroidal anti-inflammatory drug
NSTEMI: Non-ST-elevation myocardial infarction
NGT: Nasogastric tube
NO: Nitric oxide
NSR: Normal sinus rhythm
NTG: Nitroglycerin
N/V: Nausea and vomiting

N/V/D: Nausea, vomiting, diarrhea
O2: Oxygen
O2ER: Oxygen extraction ratio
OA: Osteoarthritis
Obs: Observation
OD: Overdose, oculus dextrus (right eye)
OE: On exam
OHS: Obesity hypoventilation syndrome
OM: Osteomyelitis
ONPO: Overnight pulse oximetry
OS: Oculus sinister (left eye)
OSA: Obstructive sleep apnea
OT: Occupational therapy
OTC: Over-the-counter
PaCO2: Partial pressure of carbon dioxide
PAD: Peripheral arterial disease
PAH: Pulmonary arterial hypertension
PaO2: Partial pressure of oxygen
PAP: Papanicolaou
PBW: predicted body weight
PC/AC: Pressure control/assist control
PCH: Pulmonary capillary hemangiomatosis
PCI: Percutaneous intervention
PCN: Penicillin
pCO2: Partial pressure of carbon dioxide
PCOS: Polycystic ovarian syndrome
PCP: Pneumocystis pneumonia
PCT: Procalcitonin
PCWP: Pulmonary capillary wedge pressure
PD: Parkinson's disease/personality disorder
PE: Pulmonary embolism
PEA: Pulseless electrical activity
PEEP: Positive end-expiratory pressure
PEG: Polyethylene glycol
PET: Positron emission tomography
PEx: Physical exam
P/F: PaO2/FiO2 ratio
PFO: Patent foramen ovale
PFT: Pulmonary function test
PG: Progesterone
Pheo: Pheochromocytoma
PHTN: Pulmonary hypertension
PLAX: Parasternal long axis
PLCH: Pulmonary Langerhans cell histiocytosis
PMN: Polymorphonuclear neutrophil
PNA: Pneumonia
PND: Paroxysmal nocturnal dyspnea
PO: Per oral
pO2: Partial pressure of oxygen
POCUS: Point-of-care ultrasound
POD: Post op day
PP: Post-prandial
PPD: Purified protein derivative
PPI: Proton pump inhibitor
PPM: Permanent pacemaker
PPV: Positive pressure ventilation
PRBC: Packed red blood cells
PS: Pressure support
PSA: Prostate specific antigen
PT: Physical therapy, prothrombin time
PTH: Parathyroid hormone
PTT: Partial thromboplastin time
PTSD: Post-traumatic stress disorder
PTU: Propylthiouracil
PTX: Pneumothorax
PUD: Peptic ulcer disease
PVD: Peripheral vascular disease
PVOD: Pulmonary veno-occlusive disease
PVR: Pulmonary vascular resistance
RA: Rheumatoid arthritis
RAAS: Renin angiotensin aldosterone system
Rad: Radiation
RADT: Rapid antigen detection test
RAI: Radioactive iodine
RAIU: Radioactive iodine uptake
RCC: Renal cell carcinoma
RF: Risk factor
RHD: Rheumatic heart disease
RI: Renin inhibitor
R/O: Rule out
ROSC: Return of spontaneous circulation
RPR: Rapid plasma reagin
RR: Respiratory rate
RSI: Rapid sequence induction
R/T: Related to
RTA: Renal tubular acidosis
RVSWI: Right ventricular stroke work index
R/W/S: Red/warm/swollen
Rx: Prescription/treatment
RxN: Reaction
SABA: Short-acting beta agonists
SAH: Subarachnoid hemorrhage
SAMA: Short-acting muscarinic antagonist
SBO: Small bowl obstruction
SCC: Small cell carcinoma
SCD: Sudden cardiac death, sickle cell disease
SCLC: Small cell lung cancer
SCr: Serum creatinine
ScvO2: Central venous oxygen saturation
SE: Side effect
Se: Sensitivity
SGA: Second-generation antipsychotic
SIMV: Synchronized intermittent mechanical ventilation
SJS: Stephens-Johnson syndrome
SLE: Systemic lupus erythematosus
SMA: Superior mesenteric artery
SNRI: Serotonin-norepinephrine reuptake inhibitor

SOsm: Serum osmolality
Sp: Specificity
SPEP: Serum protein electrophoresis
SpO2: oxygen saturation
SSI: Sliding scale insulin
SSRI: Selective serotonin reuptake inhibitor
SSSS: Staphylococcal scalded skin syndrome
S/T: Secondary to
STEMI: ST-elevation myocardial infarction
STI: Sexually-transmitted infection
SV: Stroke volume
SVI: Stroke volume index
SVO2: Mixed venous oxygen saturation
SVR: Stroke volume resistance
SW: Social worker
Sx: Surgery/symptom
Sz: Seizure
TACO: Transfusion-associated circulatory overload
TB: Tuberculosis
TCA: Tricyclic antidepressant
TD: Tardive dyskinesia
TDD: Total daily dose
TEN: Toxic epidermal necrolysis
TG: Triglycerides
TIPS: Transjugular intrahepatic portosystemic shunt
TM: Tympanic membrane
TMP/SMX: Trimethoprim/ sulfamethoxazole
Tmx: Trimester
TPM: Temporary pacemaker
TRALI: Transfusion-related acute lung injury
Trop: Troponin
TSH: Thyroid stimulating hormone
TT: Thrombin time
TTE: Transthoracic echocardiogram
TTP: Thrombotic thrombocytopenia purpura
TURP: Transurethral resection of the prostate
TVUS: Transvaginal ultrasound
TZD: Thiazolidinedione
UA: Urinalysis
UDS: Urine drug screen
UE: Upper extremity
UGI: Upper gastrointestinal
UGIB: Upper gastrointestinal bleed
ULN: Upper limit of normal
UNa: Urine sodium
UOP: Urinary output
UOsm: Urine osmolality
UPEP: Urine protein electrophoresis
URI: Upper respiratory tract infection
UTI: Urinary tract infection
US: Ultrasound
VBI: Vertebrobasilar insufficiency
VC/AC: Volume control/assist control
VDRL: Venereal disease research laboratory
VE: Respiratory minute volume
VF: Ventricular fibrillation
VH: Visual hallucination
VILI: Ventilation-induced lung injury
VMA: Vanillylmandelic acid
VO2: Oxygen consumption
VPA: Valproic acid
V/Q: Ventilation/perfusion
VS: Vital signs
VT: Tidal volume, ventricular tachycardia
VWD: Von Willebrand disease
WBC: White blood cell
W/D: Withdrawal
W/U: Workup

Made in the USA
Monee, IL
03 November 2026

67378306R00154